- THE WINNING -
FOOD COMBINATIONS TO PURIFY
CONTROL WEIGHT, AND
TAKE CARE OF HEALTH

PLANT - BASED
Diet after 50

**DISCOVER ALL THE
SECRETS OF A DIET
THAT CAN COUNTERACT
THE NATURAL
AGING PROCESS**

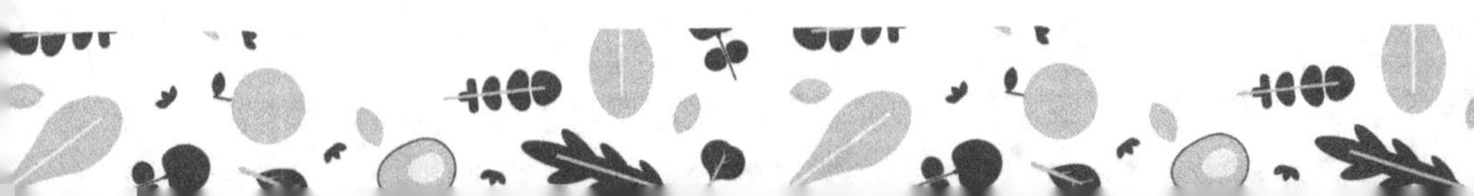

Table of *Contents*

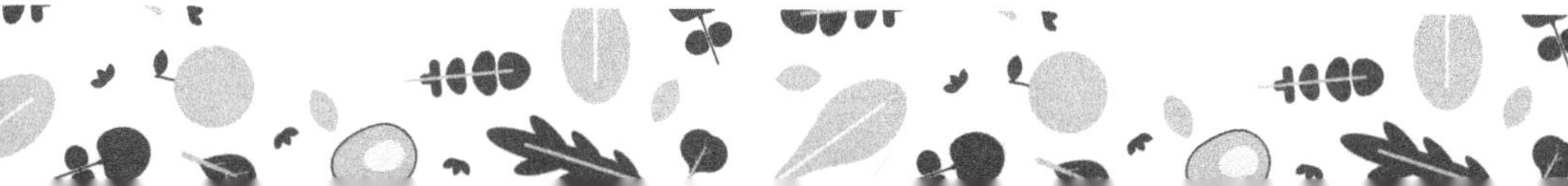

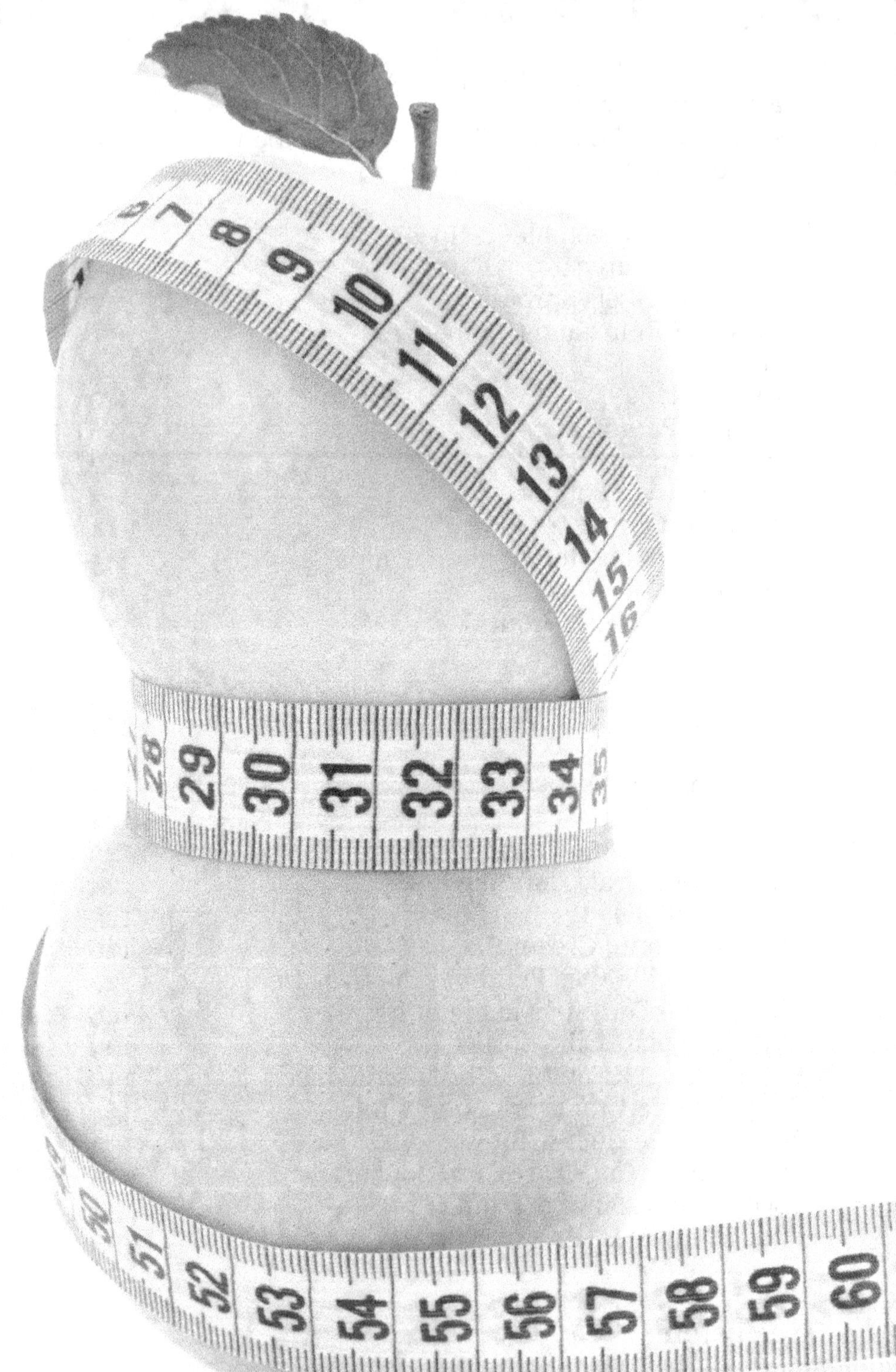

Introduction

Want a simple recipe to fight against aging? The ingredients are easy to find. The right mix of nutrients—and some regular exercise—will let you feel and look your best. When you eat right, you'll help get your weight under control, keep your bones healthy, and prevent heart disease. It's all about making smart choices.

Boost calcium and vitamin D. That means 3–4 8 oz. servings of low-fat dairy every day. If you are lactose-intolerant, eat hard cheese, yogurt, or kefir, canned salmon, broccoli, and legumes. You can also try food or drinks, like orange juice, that have the nutrients added in by the manufacturer. They'll say "fortified" on the label.

If your doctor says you do not get enough calcium in your diet, they may suggest you take supplements that have 1,000–1,500 milligrams of the nutrient.

Eat more fruits, veggies, whole grains, and legumes. These will give you plenty of disease-fighting antioxidants. Focus on variety every day, including vegetables with different colors.

Get enough fiber. You do not have to look far; some good sources are legumes, whole wheat pasta, whole grain cereals and bread, oatmeal, brown rice, popcorn, fresh fruits, and veggies.

Take a daily multivitamin. It will fill any gaps in your nutrition picture. But make sure it's tailored for your age group. When you're over 50, you need less iron than younger people.

A plant-based diet is commonly mistaken as the same as a vegetarian or vegan diet. Although these terms are often used interchangeably, they are not the same.

A plant-based diet is focused on proportionately eating more foods primarily from plants and cutting back on animal-derived foods. However, it does not necessarily involve eliminating entire food groups and lean sources of protein. It means those on a plant-based diet may still opt to eat some meat. Going vegan, on the other hand, means being strictly against animal products in any form—from never eating meat and dairy products to not patronizing products tested on animals and not wearing animal products such as leather.

A healthy plant-based diet generally emphasizes meeting your nutritional needs by eating more whole plant foods while reducing the intake of animal products. Whole foods refer to natural, unrefined, or minimally refined foods. Plant foods consist of those that do not have animal ingredients, such as meat, eggs, honey, milk, and other dairy products. In contrast, those on a vegetarian diet may still eat processed and refined foods. Vegetarians can even eat fast foods, junk food, and other salty snacks guilt-free.

Once you get started with this diet, you will notice a massive difference in how you feel each day. The moment that you wake up in the morning, you will feel that you have more energy and that you do not get tired as easily as before. You will also have more mental focus and fewer mood-related problems.

As for digestion, a plant-based diet is also said to improve how the digestive system works. Dieters confirm fewer incidences of stomach pains, bloating, indigestion, and hyperacidity.

Then there is the weight-loss benefit that we cannot forget about. Since a plant-based diet means eating fruits, vegetables, and whole grains that have fewer calories and are lower in fat, you will enjoy weight-loss benefits that some other fad diets are not able to provide.

Aside from helping you to lose weight, it maintains the ideal weight longer because this diet is easier to sustain and does not require eliminating certain food groups.

Do not worry about not getting enough nutrients from your food intake. This diet provides all the necessary nutrients, including proteins, vitamins, minerals, carbohydrates, fats, and antioxidants. And again, that is because it does not eliminate any food group but only encourages you to focus more on plant-based food products.

WHAT TO EAT AND WHAT TO AVOID?

Most people prefer to eat animal-based products for every meal. The focus of the plant-based diet plan is to make plant-based foods the primary food source. Consume animal-based foods in smaller quantities if you have a craving for them. Instead of making the animal-based foods the central part of the dish, use these foods, like seafood, meat, eggs, poultry, and dairy, as a side dish. Listed below are plant-based foods to make your choices easier:

- **Fruits:** Bananas, pears, berries, citrus fruits, pineapples, peach, etc.

- **Veggies:** Peppers, broccoli, spinach, asparagus, tomatoes, kale, carrots, cauliflower, etc.

- **Whole grains:** Rolled oats, faro, barley, quinoa, brown rice pasta, brown rice, etc.

- **Starchy veggies:** Potatoes, butternut squash, sweet potatoes, etc.

- **Legumes:** Peas, peanuts, black beans, chickpeas, lentils, etc.

- **Plant-based milk (unsweetened):** Almond milk, cashew milk, coconut milk, etc.

- **Condiments:** Mustard, lemon juice, soy sauce, salsa, nutritional yeast, vinegar, etc.

- **Nuts, nut butter, and seeds:** Pumpkin seeds, sunflower seeds, tahini, cashews, almonds, macadamia nuts, natural peanut butter (sugar-free), etc.

- **Pork and beef:** If possible, select pasture-raised or grass-fed.

- **Dairy products:** If possible, choose organic dairy products from pasture-raised animals.

- **Seafood:** If possible, pick wild-caught from sustainable fisheries.

As for foods to avoid or limit on the plant-based diet plan, the primary focus of a plant-based diet plan is to avoid as much artificially produced food as possible and add natural foods to your plate. Heavily processed foods are strictly prohibited in a plant-based diet plan. So, you must choose fresh foods while you are purchasing grocery items. Select the packaged food with the least amount of ingredients if you need to buy them necessarily. Below are listed the foods that need to be avoided on a plant-based diet plan: Added sugars and sweets like candy, soda, sugary cereals, pastries, sweet tea, table sugar, juice, cookies, etc.

The foods that must be restricted for a plant-based diet plan, even if you include healthy animal-based products in your diet are game, pork, sheep, beef, dairy, seafood, eggs, and poultry.

But let's discover more about this diet!

CHAPTER 1
What Is a Plant-Based Diet?

WHAT IS A WHOLE FOOD PLANT-BASED DIET?

The first step to following a whole food plant-based diet is understanding what it means. To put it plain and simple, it means filling a majority of your diet with foods that are not processed or refined and come directly from plants. They are foods that are as close as possible to their source and are completely unmodified. It is not a diet restricted solely to fruits and vegetables; there are many delicious alternatives to help you have a satisfying choice of foods to eat.

The benefits of a plant-based diet all depend on how an individual incorporates animal foods in their standard dietary patterns. Before you start tossing everything out of your icebox, how about we separate the details of eating a plant-based eating regimen.

GET HEALTHY WITH A PLANT-BASED DIET

Better Nutrition

Plants are very healthy foods to eat, and most people fail to eat the appropriate number of veggies and fruits, therefore, following a plant-based diet will boost your productivity. Vegetables and fruits are rich in antioxidants, vitamins, fiber, and minerals. Based on studies, fiber is a nutrient that most people do not get an adequate amount of, and it comes with tons of healthy perks—it is good for the heart, waistline, blood sugar, and the gut.

Weight-Loss

When following a plant-based diet, people tend to have a lower body mass index (BMI) than people on an omnivorous diet. However, research shows that when you follow a plant-based diet to lose weight, you will be more successful at dropping pounds and keeping them off.

Healthier Hearts

Following a plant-based diet is likely to reduce the risk of cardiovascular diseases, and enhance other heart disease risk factors by reducing cholesterol and blood pressure, and enhancing blood sugar control. Following a plant-based diet can also help quell inflammation, which increases the risk of heart disease by regulating plaque buildup in the arteries.

Lower Diabetes Risk

Irrespective of your body mass index (BMI), following a plant-based diet lowers the risk of diabetes. Another study, published in February 2019, states that you tend to have higher insulin sensitivity when you follow a plant-based diet, which is significant for maintaining a healthy blood sugar level.

Reduces the Risk of Cancer

The consistent consumption of adequate legumes, veggies, fruits, and grains is associated with lower cancer risk. However, disease-fighting phytochemicals, which can be found in plants are known to prevent and halt cancer. Lastly, studies also indicate an association between the consumption of processed meats and a rise in cancer risk, especially colorectal cancer. Therefore, there's a benefit from consuming more plants and choosing healthy plant foods rather than unhealthy ones.

GET YOUR PHYTOCHEMICALS

The only place to get phytochemicals is in whole foods, such as fruits, vegetables, beans, and whole grains. These essential nutrients have a direct impact on your health. The latest research determines that a few of the key phytochemicals might help to prevent certain cancers, lower cholesterol, keep the gastrointestinal tract healthy, and protect various cells throughout the body. There are thousands of different forms available, but the most commonly known nutrients are terms that might be a little more familiar to you: flavonoids, antioxidants, and carotenoids.

How do you fill your diet with these amazing nutrients? Start by creating a rainbow of colors on your plates. The more colorful fruits and vegetables you consume, the higher your body's chances of consuming the nutrients your body needs. There are many beautiful colored fruits and vegetables to choose from including red tomatoes, blue blueberries, orange carrots, pink watermelon, pink grapefruit, green spinach, green kale, red strawberries, and red raspberries. The more colors on your plate, the more benefits you are providing your body.

In addition to fruits and vegetables, phytonutrients can be found in whole-grain bread, whole-grain cereal, walnuts, sunflower seeds, peas, lentils, green tea, and black tea. If you consume bread and cereals, it is important to ensure that they are truly made from whole grains, not processed grains that could be stripped of the nutrients you assume you are obtaining by eating them.

IS ORGANIC A REQUIREMENT?

Eating whole foods does not mean that they must be locally grown or even organic; that is a completely different topic. This does not mean that your whole foods cannot be organic; it is just not a prerequisite to qualify as whole or natural. Organic or locally grown food could provide you with the added benefit of eliminating harmful toxins and chemicals, which can further benefit eating whole foods.

MAXIMIZE NUTRIENTS IN VEGETABLES

We eat food, besides that, it tastes good, is to obtain the vital nutrients necessary for good health. When you consume food that has been modified, processed, or refined, the important nutrients are removed. This is even true for those foods that you consider healthy. For example, you might think you are doing your body well by eating spinach or broccoli. But if you do not eat it raw or prepare it properly, you are likely losing some of its nutrients, especially water-soluble. Vitamin B and C are 2 of the water-soluble vitamins found in both vegetables that are lost when these vegetables are cooked in water, whether boiled or steamed. Choosing to eat these vegetables raw is the best way to consume all vital nutrients. If you prefer them cooked, choose methods such as sautéing, stir-frying, or blanching as each of these methods are considered "quick-cooking" methods and avoid the risk of losing many nutrients.

CHOOSING WHOLE GRAINS

In addition to eating fruits and vegetables, a whole foods diet also includes eating various whole grains. Care should be taken when you choose your grains, however. Not all whole grains are as "whole" as they sound. When you choose the right grains, you can reap the benefits of complex carbohydrates and vital vitamins and nutrients, adding taste, texture. and proper nutrition to your diet.

Grains are found in the seeds of various grasses. They can be found in various forms including wheat, oats, rice, cornmeal, and barley. When grains start, they are considered whole and their most important ingredients bran and germ are intact. During the processing of these grains, they are stripped of bran and germ as well as their vital nutrients. This results in refined and enriched grains, which make up the products that have a longer shelf life, such as white bread and white rice. These foods, as you probably know, are less healthy for you. When you read product labels, look for the words refined or enriched grains and steer clear. In refined grains, the lost nutrients are never replaced. In enriched grains, the products are fortified with the stripped nutrients, but it does not provide the same benefits as eating whole foods with the natural nutrients right from the start.

CREATING THE PERFECT MEALS

Creating the perfect meals with the right plant-based whole foods does not have to be difficult. It is best to get creative to maximize the nutrients that you consume. Start with the basics, including whole grain bread, whole grain pasta, steel-cut oats, colorful fruits, and raw vegetables. Then you can get creative:

- Add fruits and spices to your oatmeal.

- Add flaxseed to your whole-grain cereal.

- Make salad the main course for lunch or dinner and get creative.

- Add your favorite vegetables to whole grain pasta or rice.

- Make smoothies with as many fruits and vegetables as possible.

- Add plant-based, natural nut butter to whole grain bread.

- Eat fruit for dessert.

- Add beans to lunch and dinner entrées.

- Include at least one fruit and vegetable at every meal.

CHAPTER 2
What Are the Benefits of a Plant-Based Diet?

Many people mistake the plant-based diet for a vegan one. So, let's talk about the difference. There are parallels in both of them, but there are small differences. A vegan diet does not include any products based on animals. This, of course, contains meats and eggs and outcomes of these animals, such as honey. Vegans will carry this perspective into their lives, which is more than a diet to them. A plant-based diet will keep you from eating anything based on animals, but it will not prevent you from using animal products in your life.

Now that you know what the plant-based diet is, it's essential to look at the host of benefits that it has to offer. It's hard to stick to a diet that makes you drastically change your current way of eating if you do not have a good reason. That's what this chapter is about. Giving you that good reason to meet your health and weight-loss goals using the plant-based diet.

LOWERS BLOOD PRESSURE

A plant-based diet has been proven to lower blood pressure because it has a high potassium content. A plant-based diet reduces blood pressure as well as stress and anxiety. Potassium-rich foods include seeds, whole, almonds, beans, berries, and grain. However, meat contains almost no potassium, which is why the plant-based diet offers a better way to control your blood pressure.

LOWERS CHOLESTEROL

Plants do not contain cholesterol, which includes saturated forms such as coffee or chocolate. When you live a plant-based diet lifestyle, you're reducing the amount of cholesterol you take in to next to 0. This plant-based diet will lessen the danger of heart illness and disease since cholesterol is an important cause of stroke and heart attack.

MAINTAINS BLOOD SUGAR LEVELS

The plant-based diet has a lot of protein. Protein can lower blood sugar production, and in turn, it will leave you feeling full for longer. Also, a plant-based diet can reduce stress levels by lowering the cortisone levels in the body. Cortisol is a stress hormone.

STAVES OFF CHRONIC DISEASE

Chronic diseases, including diabetes, cancer, and obesity, are low in societies that follow a plant-based lifestyle. This diet has been proven to help fight off chronic disease by reducing chronic inflammation, high blood sugar, stress, and provides your body with the nutrients it needs.

WEIGHT-LOSS

In societies that follow a mainly plant-based lifestyle, obesity is also lower, which we've already covered as a chronic disease—since you're taking in more vitamins and nutrients and fiber, which your body has to break down. While you're eating a plant-based lifestyle, you're also likely to stay fuller for longer, which means you'll eat less overall. To lose weight, you have to burn more calories than you take in, so eating less is an essential part of that.

MORE ENERGY

Within days of this type of eating, you'll feel energized because you'll get the nutrients you need. The foods that you'll be eating will also have higher water content, which can hydrate your skin and leave you feeling better overall. Plant-based foods are easier to digest and lighter, so you'll feel better than ever in just a few days. You'll also get a better sleep when you eat right. When you feed your body the vitamins and minerals it needs,

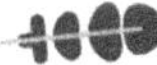

you'll help your body relax and give it a peaceful sleep. Calcium and magnesium can help relax the body for quiet rest, which this diet is packed with.

CHAPTER 3
Understanding Plant Micronutrients

Plants are rich in micronutrients that come from the soil they grow in, the basics of life they need to grow, the phytochemicals they use to protect themselves, attract insects, and adapt to the changes around them. As plants cannot move as animals do, they have a uniquely full tool chest of macro and micronutrients that enable them to adapt to the changing environment around them. These micronutrients are just as valuable to humans as they are to the plants but in different ways.

Below is a breakdown of the basic micronutrients found in fruits, vegetables, nuts, seeds, and legumes.

VITAMINS

Vibrant vegetables and fruits are a dense source of vitamins that are essential to overall health and wellness.

- **Vitamin A:** Beta-carotene is a carotenoid found in yellow, orange, and dark green fruits, and veg, most notably carrots, spinach, and broccoli. It protects against infections and is essential for eye and skin health.

- **Vitamin Bs:** This group of vitamins is responsible for maintaining the nervous system and cognitive function, DNA, and blood cell production.

  - 1 is responsible for nervous system health and aids in the breakdown and absorption of food. Found in peas, whole grains, and most fruits and vegetables.

  - 2 is responsible for energy production and healthy skin and eyes and found in asparagus, spinach, and broccoli.

  - 3 is great for healthy skin and energy production and is found in peanuts, avocados, peas, and mushrooms.

  - 4 is also essential for energy production and is found in chickpeas, potatoes, bananas, squash, and nuts.

  - 5 is also known as folate and is essential for fetal development and growth and healthy cell division. It is found in legumes, asparagus, spinach, arugula, kale, and beets.

  - 6 is predominantly sourced from animal products but you can find it in some organic soy products but most notably nutritional yeast.

- **Vitamin C:** An essential vitamin important for cell growth and energy production and tissue repair and wound healing. It is one of the most powerful antioxidants and is found in strawberries, spinach, Brussel sprouts, sweet potatoes, and tomatoes.

- **Vitamin E**: A powerful antioxidant that protects the

body from free radical damage including premature aging. It's a great support to the immune system, protecting it against external pathogens. It is found in sunflower seeds, almonds, hazelnuts, spinach, and broccoli.

- **Vitamin K:** This vitamin plays a major role in the clotting cascade and also in bone health. It is found in all green leafy veg as well as cruciferous veg and green tea.

MINERALS

Macrominerals

We need these in large quantities from our diet.

- **Calcium:** This essential mineral plays a role in bone, heart, muscle, and nerve health. Foods high in calcium are spinach, collard greens, seeds, almonds, soybeans, and butter beans.

- **Chloride:** This mineral plays a part in body fluid balance including digestive juices. It is found in sea salt, tomatoes, lettuce, celery, and rye bread.

- **Magnesium:** This mineral regulates blood sugar and assists in energy production. It also helps your muscles, kidneys, bones, and heart function effectively. It is found in spinach, quinoa, dark chocolate, almonds, avocado, and black beans.

- **Phosphorous:** This mineral is found in bones and

works with calcium in maintaining a healthy mineral balance within the body. It is found in pumpkin, sunflower seeds, lentils, chickpeas, oatmeal, and quinoa.

- **Sodium:** The current population gets excess sodium from all pre-packaged foods and restaurant meals, so there is no need to go looking for extra sodium in the diet.

- **Potassium**: This mineral is essential in blood pressure balance, muscle health, and nerve function. It is found in avocado, bananas, apricots, grapefruit, potatoes, mushrooms, cucumbers, and zucchini.

TRACE MINERALS

We just need tiny amounts of these from our foods.

- **Copper:** Essential in the formation of red blood cells and iron absorption. It is found in whole grains, beans, potatoes, cocoa, black pepper, and dark leafy greens.

- **Cobalt:** This trace mineral works closely with B12 in the formation of hemoglobin. It is found in nuts, broccoli, oats, and spinach.

- **Manganese:** Plays many roles in enzyme activity and cellular level antioxidants. It is found in pineapple, peanuts, brown rice, spinach, sweet potato, pecans, and green tea.

- **Iodine:** Essential for thyroid function, you can find it in seaweed, lima beans, and prunes.

- **Iron:** Used to make hemoglobin and as a carrier for essential nutrients in the blood. It is found in cashews, spinach, whole grains, tofu, potatoes, and lentils in plant form.

- **Selenium:** A trace mineral essential in the role of reproduction, DNA production, and antioxidant function. It is found in Brazil nuts, lentils, cashew nuts, and potatoes.

- **Zinc:** As your body does not store zinc, it needs to be consumed daily because it plays an important role in nutrient metabolism, immune system maintenance, and enzyme function. It is found in legumes, nuts, seeds, potatoes, kale, and green beans.

COLORS

The colors in fruits and vegetables point to what kinds of nutrients they contain.

- **White foods:** Contain sulfur and can have anti-cancer properties. Found in cauliflower, garlic, leeks, and onions.

- **Green foods:** Contain lutein and vitamin K. Found in dark leafy greens, broccoli, and avocado.

- **Purple foods:** Contain anthocyanins, which are powerful antioxidants. Found in blueberries, eggplant, red cabbage, and blackberries.

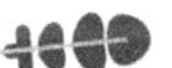
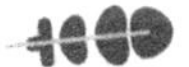

- **Red foods:** Contain lycopene and has therapeutic properties for the heart. Found in strawberries, watermelon, tomatoes, and red bell peppers.

CHAPTER 4
How Do You Start a Plant-Based Diet?

BE MENTALLY AND PSYCHOLOGICALLY READY

Eating food is a daily routine that human beings are supposed to undergo. The nature of substances and foods that we consume every day can result in a lifetime consumption habit if it is not regulated. Once the habits form, it is difficult to disband them. People surrounding us can also contribute to influencing your habits or hinder transformation. So before jumping into the plant-based lifestyle, you need to think more about it. It will help you avoid making empty promises to yourself. After you have already thought of your move to plant-based dieting, look into the obstacles that will prevent you, either psychologically or mentally, in your transformation journey. With the knowledge of the distractions, the chances of successfully getting inducted into the diet are high.

DRINK MORE WATER

Consumption of water into the body is vital. Water helps in maintaining brain health and other body operations. So, you need to replace the water that is used in the process. You should always be hydrated. The doctor here recommends taking in spring water since they are normally in an alkaline state. Tap water is often contaminated with chemicals such as chloride compounds and other chemicals.

According to the doctor, one should drink 1 gallon of spring water on a minimum daily. Avoid taking water containing softeners. Water from reverse osmosis systems should be avoided too. The work of the water is to help in nutrient absorption and organ and joint cushioning. Remember that existing health organizations do recommend the intake of 1 gallon of water as well.

You should also make the drinking of water to become a habit/culture.

INCLUDE EXTRA WHOLE MEALS TO YOUR DIET

The whole foods range from the fruits that you like to fresh fish fillets. You should distance yourself from consuming foods that are kept in packages as they are very addictive. Restraining from these foods will greatly assist you as you advance through the plant-based diet.

Work very hard in completely substituting the processed meals with whole foods. A lot of processed foods contain sugars that are enhanced. The sugars are considered very addictive as they can trigger cravings for the foods.

READ THE INGREDIENT LABELS

Avoiding other types of foods can be difficult most times. So, you can resort to reading the products' labels to know the ingredients in them. It keeps you in the know-how of what you take into your body. The habit also assists in directing you in what to change from the foods you eat. It will also assist you once you have fully embraced the diet. Here, you will be in the know of whatever you consumed.

PAY ATTENTION TO THE SNACKS

You should avoid taking packed snacks from the store.

Since you are not supposed to take packed snacks from the stores, you should stop consuming snacks. You just need to take snacks in the right way. You can try preparing some on your own. The snacks can be a mixture of raisins, walnuts, or other fruits that have been dried.

REVIEW THE APPROVED FOODS

Look into the non-recommended foods in the diet. Avoid them in every possible way that you can. When you are prepared mentally for the recommended foods, you will easily get used to them.

COOKING IS VITAL

When you have decided to follow this diet, you need to cook using the recipes recommended to you. The said guides provide people with plant-based recipes, making the technique easy to execute. The guides cover every topic in detail. As you begin meal preparation, you will learn how to use the approved ingredients for cooking the meals you like.

CHAPTER 5
Superfoods

To be clear, most superfoods are already vegan, but some are particularly high in nutrient content. The following are the top vegan superfoods available today. These should be incorporated into your diet every chance you get. The following are 12 of the best superfoods that you will find at your local grocery store.

DARK LEAFY GREENS

Kale, swiss chard, spinach, and collard greens are all classed as dark leafy greens and these superfoods should be incorporated into your daily meal plan. They are not only a great digestive aid due to their high-fiber content, but they're also dense sources of vitamins C and K, zinc, calcium, magnesium, iron, and folate. They have a high antioxidant profile that assists the body in removing harmful free radicals, reducing the risk of cancer, heart disease, and stroke.

BERRIES

These nature's little antioxidants are also the most delicious and delicate fruits we know. Berries host an array of benefits to the body and each one has its special powers:

- Strawberries contain more vitamin C than oranges! They are antioxidant-rich and provide us with fiber, potassium, anthocyanins, and folate. Strawberries reduce the risk of cancer, are supportive in the control of diabetes, and are great anti-inflammatories.

- Blueberries are one of the most antioxidant-rich foods out there. They contain manganese and vitamins C and K, are supportive of cognitive function and mental health.

- Raspberries are rich in vitamin C, selenium, and phosphorus. Research shows they are beneficial in controlling blood sugar in people with diabetes. They are a great source of quercetin known to slow the onset and growth of cancer cells.

- Blackberries are incredibly high in antioxidants and fiber and are loaded with phytochemicals that fight cancer. They are also packed with vitamin C and K.

NUTS AND SEEDS

Nuts and seeds are a vegan's best friend when it comes to texture, variety, healthy fats, and proteins. They are incredibly nutrient-dense and contain excellent levels of fats, protein, complex carbs, and fiber. They are loaded with vitamins and minerals that are easily absorbed and fun to eat, while at the same time helping to protect our bodies against disease. Every nut and seed have their special traits:

- Pine nuts have an excess amount of manganese.

- Brazil nuts are the leading source of selenium.

- Pistachios are well known for their lutein content that supports eye health.

- Almonds and sunflower seeds are great sources of vitamin E.

- Cashews have more iron than any other food in this category.

- Pumpkin seeds are one of the best possible sources of zinc.

OLIVE OIL

A staple of the Mediterranean diet for a reason, this oil is rich in antioxidants and monounsaturated fats that support cardiovascular health, prevent strokes and feed your hair and skin like nothing else. Despite being fat, it supports healthy weight maintenance.

MUSHROOMS

The best vegan meat source is low in calories while being high in protein and fiber. They're a great source of vitamins B, vitamin D, potassium, and selenium. They are high in antioxidants, support healthy gut bacteria, and are beneficial in weight-loss.

SEAWEED

Used in medicine for centuries, seaweed has antiviral properties and has recently been tested positively in killing certain cancer cells. Seaweed benefits cholesterol levels and is rich in antioxidants proven to lower the instance of heart disease. Seaweed is incredibly rich in vitamin A, C, D, E, and K, and B vitamins. It's brimming with iron and iodine, which is essential for thyroid function, and have decent amounts of calcium, copper, potassium, and magnesium.

GARLIC

Garlic is a powerful medicinal ally to have on hand. It is rich in vitamins B6 and C, but most importantly, it boosts immune function, lowers blood pressure, improves cholesterol levels, and supports cardiovascular health. Fresh garlic is brimming with antioxidants that have a potent effect on overall health.

AVOCADO

Avocado is a great source of MUFAs (Mono-Unsaturated Fatty Acids), a huge factor in cardiovascular function. They support vitamin and mineral absorption, healthy skin, hair, and eyes, improved digestive function, and contain 20 vitamins and minerals. Avocados provide anti-inflammatory activity and are loaded with soluble fiber.

TURMERIC

Highly anti-inflammatory and has potent anti-cancer properties. It has been shown to provide pain relief in arthritic conditions and supports liver health due to its high antioxidant levels. Turmeric can be hard to absorb, however, taking it with black pepper improves its absorptivity.

CHIA SEEDS

These tiny seeds are packed full of omega 3 fatty acids, they are one of the best vegan sources out there. They are also antioxidant-rich and packed with protein, calcium, iron, and soluble fiber. Due to this, they are recommended to reduce cardiovascular disease, diabetes, and obesity. They are healing to the digestive tract, contribute to feelings of fullness so support weight-loss, help lower cholesterol, and best of all, when mixed with water, they make a great egg substitute.

LEGUMES

A study was conducted that investigated the longest living people and cultures in the world. The only dietary thing they shared was that legumes were a huge part of their diet, in fact, the longest living people in the world eat them every day. Legumes are rich in protein, fiber, and complex carbohydrates, and contain potassium, magnesium, folate, iron, B vitamins, zinc, copper, manganese, and phosphorus. These little guys are highly nutritious and loaded with soluble fiber that benefits colon health, feed healthy bacteria, and reduce the risk of colon cancer.

CHAPTER 6
Looking for Alternatives

Here are some tips to get you started so you can stick to this diet with ease!

LOOK FOR MILK ALTERNATIVES

There are many non-dairy milk alternatives out there. There is coconut, cashew, Brazil nut, rice, almond, and even hemp seed milk substitutes. Most can be used in equal measurements, especially in baking. Just make sure you're using their unsweetened versions. The best is that most of these kinds of milk are rich in calcium so you won't be missing out.

LOOK FOR EGG ALTERNATIVES

You can also replace eggs in recipes. You can use 6 tbsps. of water with 3 tbsps. of chia seeds or ground flaxseeds. Just soak them for 5–10 minutes so that the mixture becomes gelatinous. You can also use ¼ c. of pureed

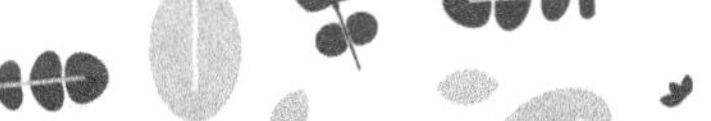
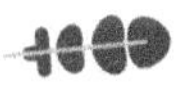

banana or ¼ c. of applesauce. Depending on the recipe. Each one of these is the equivalent of 1 single egg.

LOOK FOR CHEESE ALTERNATIVES

There isn't a substitute for cheese, but the plant world has soft and creamy textures that can make cheese. It does make a small change in the dish's taste, but it isn't too bad. The most popular replacements are soaked and blended cashews, sliced avocado, sprouted soft organic tofu, and nutritional yeast.

LOOK FOR MEAT ALTERNATIVES

For a rich, hearty texture that will help fill you up, there are beans, Portobello mushrooms, tempeh, and tofu. Each of these is chewy and hearty, and they can be marinated to get different flavors. You can also use these for chili, stews, and burgers, or can be served baked.

BE CAREFUL EATING OUT

It can be hard to dine out when you're trying to enjoy a plant-based diet. However, many restaurants offer vegan options, so try to look for one in advance. Just realize that you'll need to minimize the number of times you eat out. However, if you need to go out, then check out the menu online before you arrive. Look for dishes that are low in fat and full of vegetables, and then look for grilled, baked, and steamed options. Try to avoid any dishes that are fried, rich, creamy, or crispy. Just do not be shy about asking for a different salad dressing or side dish either. Make sure sauces and cheeses are left out too. If there's bread, ask for whole wheat. If there is rice, ask for brown rice.

PURGE YOUR KITCHEN

You should get rid of any temptation that's in your kitchen and calling your name if you're trying to start a plant-based diet. It's not good to have unhealthy foods in front of you, or you're bound to give in.

PLAN YOUR MEALS

Luckily this book comes with a meal plan that will help you stick to your first 3 weeks of your diet. However, you may want to stick to planning your meals for the first few months if you find yourself struggling.

CHOOSE THE ONE FOR YOU

You can choose the plant-based diet for you! Here are some of the most common plant-based diets out there:

- **Veganism:** This is a diet that includes legumes, fruits, grains, vegetables, nuts, and seeds, but you'll not be able to eat any food that's sourced from animals.

- **Raw Veganism:** This is a diet that includes uncooked and some dehydrated foods.

- **Vegetarianism:** This is a diet that consists of legumes, vegetables, nuts, and fruit. You can include eggs and dairy in this diet, but you aren't allowed meat.

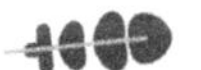
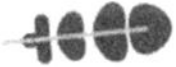

- **Fruitarianism:** This is a vegan diet that primarily involves fruit, but you should not use this if you have diabetes.

- **Ovo-Lacto Vegetarianism:** This encourages that you eat eggs and dairy along with your fruit and vegetables.

- **Ovo Vegetarianism:** This is where you can eat eggs with your fruits and vegetables, but you still can't have dairy.

- **Lacto Vegetarianism:** This allows you to have dairy but no eggs with your fruits and vegetables.

- **Semi-Vegetarianism:** This is a mostly vegetarian diet with the occasional time that you can have meat.

- **Pescatarian:** This is a semi-vegetarian diet that allows you to have dairy, eggs, shellfish, and fish.

- **Macrobiotic Diet:** This diet highlights whole grains, beans, miso soup, sea vegetables, vegetables, and naturally processed foods. This can be done with or without seafood and other animal products.

CHAPTER 7
Shopping List

The freezer is one of the most useful devices when meal shopping preparation, but to make life easier there are some things to keep in mind:

- It is a good idea to clean out your freezer regularly.

- Store your food at room temperature or in the refrigerator before freezing so that your food is not hot when you put it in-which thaws the ice and food around it.

- Keeping the freezer full is more economical and air will be kept cold more easily but do not overload it so that no air can circulate.

- Be careful not to keep the door open for long when taking food in and out as the food inside will start to defrost and go bad.

SAMPLE SHOPPING LIST

- 1 green apple
- 2 packages of coconut milk
- 1 package of cinnamon
- 1 package of salt
- 1 package of pepper
- 1 package of vegan protein powder, vanilla flavored
- 1 package of vegan protein powder, chocolate flavored
- 1 bottle of olive oil
- 1 package of coconut oil
- 2 packages of chia seeds
- 2 packages of pecans
- 2 packages of raw cashews
- 1 package of dates
- 2 lemons
- 1 package of portobello mushrooms
- 2 potatoes
- 3 avocados
- 1 package of cilantro
- 1 package of tomatoes
- 1 red onion
- 1 jalapeño
- 1 package of whole wheat flour
- 1 bottle of maple syrup
- 1 package of miso paste, yellow or white
- 1 package of sesame oil
- 1 package of chickpeas
- 1 package of green or brown lentils
- 1 package of silken tofu
- 2 radishes
- 3 cherry tomatoes
- 1 package of sesame seeds
- 1 package of gluten-free noodles
- 1 package of almond flour
- 1 package of tamari sauce
- 1 package of tomato paste
- 1 package of mushrooms
- 1 package of thyme

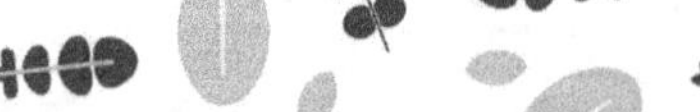
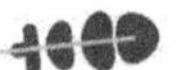

- 2 packages of spinach
- 1 bottle of apple cider vinegar
- 3 packages of almonds
- 2 packages of walnuts
- 1 package of nutmeg
- 1 package of cashew butter
- 5 bananas
- 2 packages of oats
- 1 package of pure vanilla extract
- 1 package of almond milk
- 2 butternut squashes
- 1 package of broccoli
- 1 package of French green lentils
- 1 head of garlic
- 1 package of onion powder
- 1 package of cumin
- 1 package of paprika
- 1 package of oregano
- 1 package of red pepper flakes
- 2 purple onions
- 1 jar of applesauce
- 1 package of baking powder
- 2 zucchinis
- 2 packages of quinoa
- 1 pineapple
- 1 ginger root
- 2 white onions
- 2 green bell peppers
- 1 red bell peppers
- 1 bottle of rice vinegar
- 1 package of low-sodium soy sauce
- 2 packages of extra-firm tofu, drained
- 1 package of cornstarch
- 1 package of coconut sugar
- 1 package of carob chips
- 1 package of puffy rice cereal
- 1 package of almond butter
- 1 package of flaxseeds

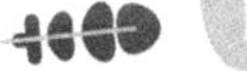
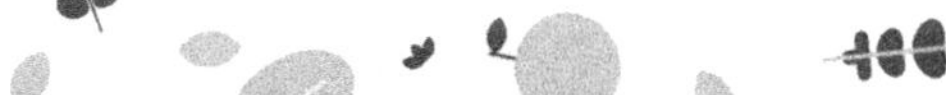

- 1 package of onion flakes
- 1 package of peanuts
- 1 package of garbanzo beans
- 1 package of golden raisins
- 1 package of turmeric
- 2 eggplants, large
- 1 package of allspice
- 1 package of tomato sauce
- 1 package of sweet onions
- 1 package cocoa powder
- 1 package of agave nectar
- 1 package of brewed coffee
- 1 package of black beans
- 2 packages of tempeh
- 1 lime
- 1 large bunch of kale
- 1 package of oat milk
- 1 package of sunflower butter
- 2 heirloom tomatoes
- 1 package of fennel seeds
- 1 yellow squash
- 1 package of basil
- 2 cans of chickpeas
- 1 package of garlic powder
- 1 package of cayenne
- 1 package of collard greens
- 1 package of gluten-free grits
- 1 package of smoked paprika
- 1 package of peanut butter
- 1 package of shredded coconut
- 1 package of dried cranberries
- 1 package of navy beans
- 1 package of rice, of choice
- 1 sweet potato

CHAPTER 8
Breakfast

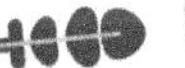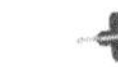

Preparation: 30' **Cooking:** 20' **Servings:** 6

GINGERBREAD WAFFLES

INGREDIENTS

- 1 c. spelt flour
- 2 tsps. baking powder
- ¼ tsp. salt
- 1 tbsp. ground flaxseeds
- 1 ½ tsps. ground cinnamon
- 2 tsps. ground ginger
- 4 tbsps. coconut sugar
- ¼ tsp. baking soda
- 1 ½ tbsps. olive oil
- 1 c. non-dairy milk
- 1 tbsp. apple cider vinegar
- 2 tbsps. blackstrap molasses

DIRECTIONS

1. Take a waffle iron, oil generously, and preheat.
2. Take a large bowl and add the dry ingredients. Stir well together.
3. Put the wet ingredients into another bowl and stir until combined.
4. Stir the dry and wet together until combined.
5. Pour the mixture into the waffle iron and cook at medium temperature for 20 minutes.
6. Open carefully and remove.
7. Serve and enjoy.

NUTRITION

Calories: 173.
Fat: 5 g.

Carbohydrates: 29 g.
Protein: 3 g.

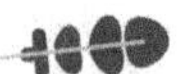
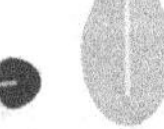
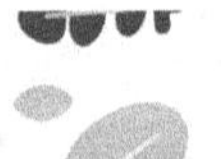
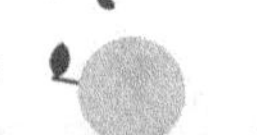
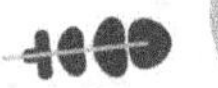

Preparation: 20'   **Cooking:** 25'   **Servings:** 12

BLUEBERRY FRENCH TOAST BREAKFAST MUFFINS

INGREDIENTS

- 1 c. unsweetened plant milk
- 1 tbsp. ground flaxseed
- 1 tbsp. almond meal
- 1 tbsp. maple syrup
- 1 tsp. vanilla extract
- 1 tsp. cinnamon
- 2 tsps. nutritional yeast
- ¾ c. frozen blueberries
- 9 slices soft bread, each cut into 4
- ¼ c. oats
- ⅓ c. raw pecans
- ¼ c. of coconut sugar
- 3 tbsps. coconut butter, at room temperature
- ⅛ tsp. sea salt

DIRECTIONS

1. Preheat your oven to 370°F and grease a muffin tin. Pop to one side.
2. Find a medium bowl and add the flaxseeds, almond meal, nutritional yeast, maple syrup, milk, vanilla, and cinnamon.
3. Mix well using a fork, then pop into the fridge.
4. Grab your food processor and add the topping ingredients (except the coconut butter). Whizz to combine.
5. Add the butter, then whizz again.
6. Grab your muffin tin and add 1 tsp. of the flax and cinnamon batter to the bottom of each space.
7. Add a square of the bread, then top with 5–6 blueberries.
8. Sprinkle with 2 tsps. of the crumble, then top with another piece of bread.
9. Place 5–6 more blueberries over the bread, sprinkle with more of the topping, then add the other piece of bread.
10. Add 1 tbsp. of the flax and cinnamon mixture over the top and add a couple of blueberries on the top.
11. Pop into the oven and cook for 20–25 minutes until the top begins to brown. Serve and enjoy.

NUTRITION

Calories: 132.   Carbohydrates: 14 g.
Fat: 5 g.   Protein: 3 g.

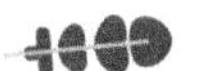

Preparation: 25'   **Cooking:** 5'   **Servings:** 2

GREEK GARBANZO BEANS ON TOAST

INGREDIENTS

- 2 tbsps. olive oil
- 3 small shallots, finely diced
- 2 large garlic cloves, finely diced
- ¼ tsp. smoked paprika
- ½ tsp. sweet paprika
- ½ tsp. cinnamon
- ½ tsp. salt
- ½–1 tsp. sugar, to taste
- Black pepper, to taste
- 1 (14 oz.) can peel plum tomatoes
- 2 c. cooked garbanzo beans
- 4–6 slices of crusty bread, toasted
- Fresh parsley and dill
- Pitted Kalamata olives

DIRECTIONS

1. Put a skillet over medium heat and add the oil.
2. Add the shallots to the pan and cook for 5 minutes.
3. Add the garlic and cook until ready, then add the other spices to the pan.
4. Stir well, then add the tomatoes.
5. Lower the heat and simmer on low until the sauce thickens.
6. Add the garbanzo beans and warm through.
7. Season with sugar, salt, and pepper, then serve and enjoy.

NUTRITION

Calories: 709.
Fat: 12 g.

Carbohydrates: 23 g.
Protein: 19 g.

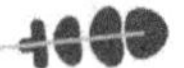

Preparation: 5'   Cooking: 12'   Servings: 1

FLUFFY GARBANZO BEAN OMELET

INGREDIENTS

- ¼ c. besan flour
- 1 tbsp. nutritional yeast
- ½ tsp. baking powder
- ¼ tsp. turmeric
- ½ tsp. chopped chives
- ¼ tsp. garlic powder
- ⅛ tsp. black pepper
- ½ tsp. Ener-G egg replacer
- ¼ c. + 1 tbsp. water
- Leafy greens, torn with hands
- Veggies
- Salsa
- Ketchup
- Hot sauce
- Parsley

DIRECTIONS

1. Grab a medium bowl and combine all the ingredients, except the greens and veggies. Leave to stand for 5 minutes.
2. Place a skillet over medium heat and add the oil.
3. Pour the batter into the pan, spread, and cook for 3–5 minutes until the edges pull away from the pan.
4. Add the greens and the veggies of your choice, then fold the omelet over.
5. Cook for 2 more minutes, then put it onto a plate.
6. Serve with the topping of your choice.
7. Serve and enjoy.

NUTRITION

Calories: 439.
Fat: 8 g.

Carbohydrates: 35 g.
Protein: 12 g.

Preparation: 10'   Cooking: 10'   Servings: 1

EASY HUMMUS TOAST

INGREDIENTS

- 2 slices of sprouted wheat bread
- ¼ c. hummus
- 1 tbsp. hemp seeds
- 1 tbsp. roasted unsalted sunflower seeds

DIRECTIONS

1. Start by toasting your bread.
2. Top with the hummus and seeds, then eat!

NUTRITION

Calories: 316.
Fat: 16 g.

Carbohydrates: 13 g.
Protein: 18 g.

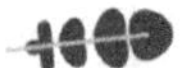
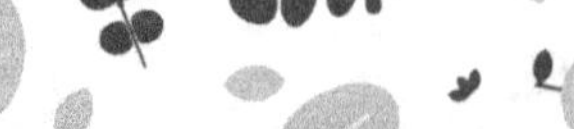
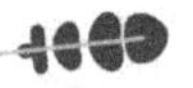

Preparation: 10'   **Cooking:** 10'   **Servings:** 8

NO-BAKE CHEWY GRANOLA BARS

INGREDIENTS

- ¼ tsp. cinnamon
- ¼ tsp. salt
- ½ tsp. cardamom
- ¼ c. of coconut oil
- 1 c. oats
- 1 tsp. vanilla extract
- ½ c. raw almonds, sliced
- ¼ c. sunflower seeds
- ½ c. pumpkin seeds
- 1¼ tsp. nutmeg
- 1 tbsp. chia seeds
- ¼ c. honey
- 1 c. dried figs, chopped

DIRECTIONS

1. Line a 6" x 8" baking dish with parchment paper and place it to one side.
2. Grab a saucepan and add the salt, honey, oil, and spices.
3. Place over medium heat and stir until it melts together.
4. Reduce the heat, add the oats, and stir.
5. Add the dried fruit, seeds, and nuts, and stir through again.
6. Cook for 10 minutes.
7. Remove from the heat and transfer the oat mixture to the pan.
8. Press down until it's packed firm.
9. Let it to cool completely, then cut into 8 bars.
10. Serve and enjoy.

NUTRITION

Calories: 308.
Fat: 14 g.

Carbohydrates: 35 g.
Protein: 6 g.

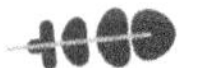
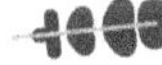

Preparation: 5'   Cooking: 10'   Servings: 2

TASTY OATMEAL AND CARROT CAKE

INGREDIENTS

- 1 c. of water
- ½ tsp. of cinnamon
- 1 c. of rolled oats
- Salt
- ¼ c. of raisins
- ½ c. of shredded carrots
- 1 c. of non-dairy milk
- ¼ tsp. of allspice
- ½ tsp. of vanilla extract

For the toppings:

- ¼ c. of chopped walnuts
- 2 tbsps. of maple syrup
- 2 tbsps. of shredded coconut

DIRECTIONS

1. Put a small pot on low heat and bring the non-dairy milk, oats, and water to a simmer.
2. Now, add the carrots, vanilla extract, raisins, salt, cinnamon, and allspice. You need to simmer all the ingredients, but do not forget to stir them. You will know that they are ready when the liquid is fully absorbed into all the ingredients (in about 7–10 minutes).
3. Transfer the thickened dish to bowls. You can top them with coconut or walnuts.
4. This nutritious bowl will allow you to kick-start your day.

NUTRITION

Calories: 210.   Carbohydrates: 42 g.
Fat: 11 g.   Protein: 4 g.

Preparation: 5'   Cooking: 10'   Servings: 2

ALMOND BUTTER BANANA OVERNIGHT OATS

INGREDIENTS

- ½ c. rolled oats
- 1 c. almond milk
- 1 tbsp. chia seeds
- ¼ tsp. vanilla extract
- ½ tsp. ground cinnamon
- 1 tbsp. honey or maple syrup
- 1 banana, sliced
- 2 tbsps. natural almond butter

DIRECTIONS

1. Take a large bowl and add the oats, milk, chia seeds, vanilla, cinnamon, and honey.
2. Stir to combine, then divide half of the mixture between 2 bowls.
3. Top with the banana and peanut butter, then add the remaining mixture.
4. Cover then, put into the fridge overnight.
5. Serve and enjoy.

NUTRITION

Calories: 227.
Fat: 11 g.

Carbohydrates: 35 g.
Protein: 7 g.

Preparation: 5'   **Cooking:** 10'   **Servings:** 4

PEACH AND CHIA SEED BREAKFAST PARFAIT

INGREDIENTS

- ¼ c. chia seeds
- 1 tbsp. pure maple syrup
- 1 c. of coconut milk
- 1 tsp. ground cinnamon
- 3 medium peaches, diced small
- ⅔ c. granola

DIRECTIONS

1. Find a small bowl and add the chia seeds, maple syrup, and coconut milk.
2. Stir well, then cover and put into the fridge for at least 1 hour.
3. Find another bowl, add the peaches and sprinkle with the cinnamon. Put them to one side.
4. When it's time to serve, take 2 glasses, and pour the chia mixture between the 2.
5. Sprinkle the granola over the top, keeping a tiny amount to one side to use to decorate later.
6. Top with the peaches and the reserved granola and serve.

NUTRITION

Calories: 260.
Fat: 13 g.

Carbohydrates: 22 g.
Protein: 6 g.

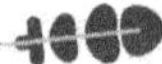

Preparation: 5' Cooking: 6' Servings: 4

AVOCADO TOAST WITH WHITE BEANS

INGREDIENTS

- ½ c. canned white beans, drained and rinsed
- 2 tsps. tahini paste
- 2 tsps. lemon juice
- ½ tsp. salt
- ½ avocado, peeled and pit removed
- 4 slices whole grain bread, toasted
- ½ c. grape tomatoes, cut in half

DIRECTIONS

1. In a small bowl, add the beans, tahini, juice of ½ lemon, and ½ tsp. of salt. Mash with a fork.
2. Take another bowl and add the avocado, the remaining lemon juice, and the salt. Mash together.
3. Place your toast onto a flat surface and add the mashed beans, spreading well.
4. Top with the avocado and the sliced tomatoes, then serve and enjoy.

NUTRITION

Calories: 140.
Fat: 5 g.

Carbohydrates: 13 g.
Protein: 5 g.

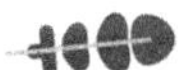
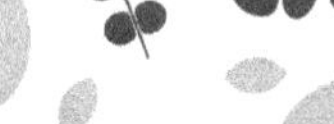
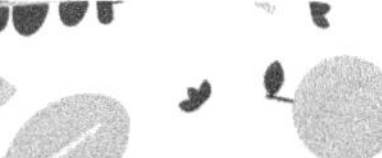
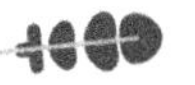

Preparation: 10'   Cooking: 0'   Servings: 8

OATMEAL AND PEANUT BUTTER BREAKFAST BAR

INGREDIENTS

- 1 ½ c. date, pit removed
- ½ c. peanut butter
- ½ c. old-fashioned rolled oats

DIRECTIONS

1. Grease a baking tin and put to one side.
2. In your food processor, add the dates, and whizz until chopped.
3. Add the peanut butter and the oats and pulse.
4. Scoop into the baking tin, then put into the fridge or freezer until set.
5. Serve and enjoy.

NUTRITION

Calories: 232.
Fat: 9 g.

Carbohydrates: 32 g.
Protein: 8 g.

CHAPTER 9

Mains

Preparation: 5'   Cooking: 30'   Servings: 8

ORANGE FRENCH TOAST

INGREDIENTS

- 2 c. of plant milk (unflavored)
- 4 tbsps. maple syrup
- 1 ½ tbsps. cinnamon
- Salt (optional)
- 1 c. almond flour
- 1 tbsp. orange zest
- 8 bread slices

DIRECTIONS

1. Turn on the oven and heat to 400°F afterward.
2. In a cup, add the ingredients and whisk until the batter is smooth.
3. Dip each piece of bread into the paste and let it soak for a couple of seconds.
4. Put it in the pan, and cook until lightly browned.
5. Put the toast on the cookie sheet and bake for 10–15 minutes in the oven, until it is crispy.

NUTRITION

Calories: 129.   Carbohydrates: 21.5 g.
Fat: 1.1 g.   Protein: 7.9 g.

Preparation: 5'   **Cooking:** 30'   **Servings:** 8

CHOCOLATE CHIP COCONUT PANCAKES

INGREDIENTS

- 1 ¼ c. oats
- 2 tsps. coconut flakes
- 2 c. plant milk
- 1 ¼ c. maple syrup
- 1 ⅓ c. of chocolate chips
- 2 ¼ c. buckwheat flour
- 2 tsps. baking powder
- 1 tsp. vanilla essence
- 2 tsps. flaxseed meal
- Salt (optional)
- ¼ c. flour
- 2 tbsp. sugar

DIRECTIONS

1. Put the flaxseed and cook over medium heat until the paste becomes a little moist.
2. Remove seeds.
3. Stir the buckwheat, oats, coconut, chips, baking powder, and salt with each other in a wide dish.
4. In a large dish, stir together the reserved flax water with the sugar, maple syrup, vanilla essence.
5. Transfer the wet mixture to the dry ingredients and shake to combine
6. Place the nonstick grill pan over medium heat.
7. Pour ¼ c. flour onto the grill pan with each pancake, and scatter gently.
8. Cook for 5–6 minutes, before the pancakes appear somewhat crispy.

NUTRITION

Calories: 198.
Fat: 9.1 g.

Carbohydrates: 11.5 g.
Protein: 7.9 g.

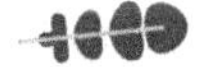

Preparation: 10'   **Cooking:** 30'   **Servings:** 3

CHICKPEA OMELET

INGREDIENTS

- 2 c. flour (chickpea)
- 1 ½ tsps. onion powder
- 1 ½ tsps. garlic powder
- ¼ tsp. pepper (white and black)
- ⅓ c. yeast
- 1 tsp. baking powder
- 3 green onions (chopped)
- 1 c. sugar
- 1 c. mushrooms

DIRECTIONS

1. In a bowl, add the chickpea flour and spices.
2. Apply 1 c. of sugar, then stir.
3. Power medium-heat and put the frying pan.
4. On each omelet, add onions and mushrooms in the batter while it heats.
5. Serve your delicious Chickpea Omelet.

NUTRITION

Calories: 399.
Fat: 11.1 g.

Carbohydrates: 11.5 g.
Protein: 7.9 g.

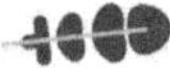

Preparation: 5'   Cooking: 15'   Servings: 1-2

APPLE-LEMON BOWL

INGREDIENTS

- 6 apples
- 3 tbsps. walnuts
- 7 dates
- Lemon juice
- ½ tsp. cinnamon

DIRECTIONS

1. Root the apples, then break them into wide bits.
2. In a bowl, put dates, part of the lemon juice, walnuts, cinnamon, and ¾ of the apples. Thinly slice until finely ground.
3. Apply the remaining apples and lemon juice and make slices.

NUTRITION

Calories: 249.
Fat: 5.1 g.

Carbohydrates: 71.5 g.
Protein: 7.9 g.

Preparation: 10'   **Cooking:** 30'   **Servings:** 6

BREAKFAST SCRAMBLE

INGREDIENTS

- 1 red onion
- 2 tbsps. soy sauce
- 2 c. sliced mushrooms
- Salt to taste
- 1 ½ tsps. black pepper
- 1 ½ tsps. turmeric
- ¼ tsp. cayenne
- 3 cloves garlic
- 1 red bell pepper
- 1 large head cauliflower
- 1 green bell pepper

DIRECTIONS

1. In a small pan, put all vegetables and cook until crispy.
2. Stir in the cauliflower and cook for 4–6 minutes or until it smooths.
3. Add spices to the pan and cook for another 5 minutes.

NUTRITION

Calories: 199.
Fat: 1.1 g.

Carbohydrates: 14.5 g.
Protein: 7.9 g.

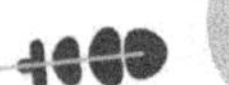

Preparation: 5' Cooking: 15' Servings: 4

BROWN RICE BREAKFAST PUDDING

INGREDIENTS

- 2 c. almond milk
- 1 c. dates, chopped
- 1 apple, chopped
- Salt to taste
- ¼ c. almonds, toasted
- 1 cinnamon stick
- Ground cloves to taste
- 3 c. cooked rice
- 1 tbsp. raisins

DIRECTIONS

1. Calories: 299.
2. Fat: 1.1 g.
3. Carbohydrates: 71.5 g.
4. Protein: 7.9 g.

NUTRITION

Calories: 132.
Fat: 5 g.

Carbohydrates: 14 g.
Protein: 3 g.

Preparation: 10'   Cooking: 30'   Servings: 4

BLACK BEAN AND SWEET POTATO HASH

INGREDIENTS

- 1 c. onion, chopped
- ⅓ c. vegetable broth
- 2 garlic, minced
- 1 c. cooked black beans
- 2 tsps. hot chili powder
- 2 c. chopped sweet potatoes
- 1 tbsp. green onion chopped

DIRECTIONS

1. Put the onions in a saucepan over medium heat and add the seasoning, and mix.
2. Add potatoes and chili, then mix.
3. Cook for around 12 minutes more until the vegetables are cooked thoroughly.
4. Add the green onion, beans, and salt.
5. Cook for 2 minutes more and serve.

NUTRITION

Calories: 239.
Fat: 1.1 g.

Carbohydrates: 71.5 g.
Protein: 7.9 g.

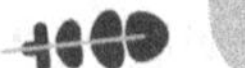
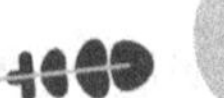
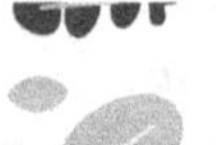
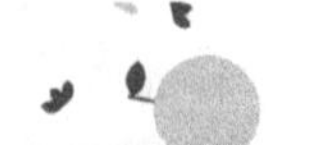
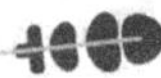

Preparation: 15' **Cooking**: 60' **Servings**: 8

APPLE-WALNUT BREAKFAST BREAD

INGREDIENTS

- 1 ½ c. apple sauce
- ⅓ c. plant milk
- 2 c. all-purpose flour
- Salt to taste
- 1 tsp. ground cinnamon
- 1 tbsp. flaxseeds mixed with 2 tbsps. warm water
- ¾ c. brown sugar
- 1 tsp. baking powder
- ¼ cup walnuts

DIRECTIONS

1. Preheat to 375°F.
2. Combine the apple sauce, sugar, milk, and flax mixture in a jar and mix.
3. Combine the flour, baking powder, salt, walnuts, and cinnamon in a separate bowl.
4. Simply add the dry ingredients into the wet ingredients and combine them to make slices.
5. Bake for 25 minutes until it becomes light brown.

NUTRITION

Calories: 309.
Fat: 9.1 g.

Carbohydrates: 16.5 g.
Protein: 6.9 g.

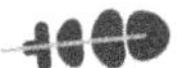

Preparation: 10'   **Cooking:** 30'   **Servings:** 2

VEGAN SALMON BAGEL

INGREDIENTS

- Salt and pepper
- 1 ½ c. of apple cider vinegar
- 7 carrots
- 1 tbsp. sugar

DIRECTIONS

1. Preheat to 200°C.
2. Slice the carrots.
3. In a mixer to mix, combine sugar, vinegar, and ground pepper.
4. Put the carrot strips in a stir fry bowl, apply the marinade, and stir.
5. Cover the carrots with foil and bake for 20 minutes, then switch heat down to 210°F and cook for 40 minutes more.

NUTRITION

Calories: 232.
Fat: 9.1 g.

Carbohydrates: 71.5 g.
Protein: 7.9 g.

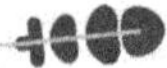

Preparation: 5' | Cooking: 10' | Servings: 1

MINT CHOCOLATE GREEN PROTEIN SMOOTHIE

INGREDIENTS

- 1 scoop chocolate powder
- 1 tbsp. flaxseed
- 1 banana
- 1 mint leaf
- ¾ c. almond milk
- 3 tbsps. dark chocolate (chopped)

DIRECTIONS

1. Blend all the ingredients, except the dark chocolate.
2. Garnish with dark chocolate when ready.

NUTRITION

Calories: 300.
Fat: 19.1 g.

Carbohydrates: 21.5 g.
Protein: 27.9 g.

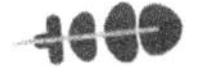

Preparation: 5' Cooking: 10' Servings: 2

DAIRY-FREE COCONUT YOGURT

INGREDIENTS

- 1 can coconut milk
- 4 vegan probiotic capsules

DIRECTIONS

1. Shake coconut milk with a whole tube.
2. Remove the plastic of the capsules and mix in.
3. Cut a 12-inch cheesecloth until stirred.
4. Freeze or eat immediately.

NUTRITION

Calories: 219.
Fat: 10.1 g.

Carbohydrates: 1.5 g.
Protein: 7.9 g.

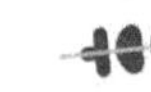

Preparation: 5'   Cooking: 10'   Servings: 2

VEGAN GREEN AVOCADO SMOOTHIE

INGREDIENTS

- 1 banana
- 1 c. water
- ½ avocado
- ½ lemon juice
- ½ c. coconut yogurt

DIRECTIONS

1. Blend all ingredients until smooth.

NUTRITION

Calories: 299.
Fat: 1.1 g.

Carbohydrates: 1.5 g.
Protein: 7.9 g.

Preparation: 10'　　　**Cooking:** 35'　　　**Servings:** 12

SUN-BUTTER BAKED OATMEAL CUPS

INGREDIENTS

- ¼ c. coconut sugar
- 1 ½ rolled oats
- 2 tbsps. chia seeds
- ¼ tsp. salt
- 1 tsp. cinnamon
- ½ c. non-dairy milk
- ½ c. Sun-Butter
- ½ c. apple sauce

DIRECTIONS

1. Preheat the oven to 350°F.
2. Mix all ingredients and blend well.
3. Add in muffin cups and insert extra toppings.
4. Bake 25 minutes, or until golden brown.

NUTRITION

Calories: 129.　　　　Carbohydrates: 1.5 g.
Fat: 1.1 g.　　　　　　Protein: 4.9 g.

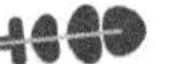

Preparation: 5'   Cooking: 5'   Servings: 2

CHOCOLATE PEANUT BUTTER SHAKE

INGREDIENTS

- 2 bananas
- 3 tbsps. peanut butter
- 1 c. almond milk
- 3 tbsps. cacao powder

DIRECTIONS

1. Combine ingredients in a blender.
2. Blend them until smooth.

NUTRITION

Calories: 149.
Fat: 1.1 g.

Carbohydrates: 1.5 g.
Protein: 7.9 g.

CHAPTER 10
Snack and Side Recipes

Preparation: 6'   **Cooking:** 35'   **Servings:** 6

SAUSAGE ROLLS

INGREDIENTS

- 2 slices whole-wheat bread
- ½ c. mixed nuts, halves, and in pieces
- 2 tbsps. cranberries, dried
- 1 ½ tsps. sea salt
- 1 tsp. thyme, fresh and chopped
- 1 tsp. sage, dried
- 1 tsp. smoked paprika
- 1 tsp. sweet paprika
- ¼ tsp. ground black pepper
- 1 ½ tbsps. tamari sauce
- 1 tsp. sriracha
- 2 tbsps. aquafaba egg replacement
- 10 oz. tofu, firm
- 3 prepared sheets vegan puff pastry

DIRECTIONS

1. Preheat your large baking oven to a temperature of 375°F and prepare a large sheet for baking with either non-stick silicone or kitchen parchment.
2. In a large food processor, pulse together the sliced bread, mixed nuts, cranberries, and herbs until they form a fine meal or crumb.
3. In the food processor, along with the bread and nut mixture, add the tofu, sea salt, tamari sauce, sriracha, aquafaba, ground black pepper, and both the smoked and sweet paprika. Pulse this mixture until it is well combined, stirring the container's sides with a spatula as needed. Set this aside.
4. Lay out the 3 prepared sheets of puff pastry on a cutting board and slice each sheet into 4 evenly-sized squares so that you end up with 12 squares in all.
5. Divide the tofu sausage mixture between the 12 squares, placing the mixture in each puff pastry piece's center. Roll the squares up so that the puff pastry completely contains the filling.
6. Using a sharp knife, cut each of the 12 rolls in half so that you end up with 24 smaller sausage rolls. Place all 24 sausage rolls on the prepared baking tray with the puff pastry's seam side facing downward. This will prevent the filling from falling out during the cooking process.
7. Place the sausage rolls in the oven until the puff pastry is golden, about 20–25 minutes. Serve the rolls alone or with your favorite complimentary chutney.

NUTRITION

Calories: 308.
Protein: 13 g.
Fat: 18 g.

Total carbohydrates: 25 g.
Net carbohydrates: 22 g.

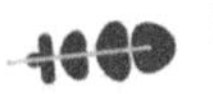
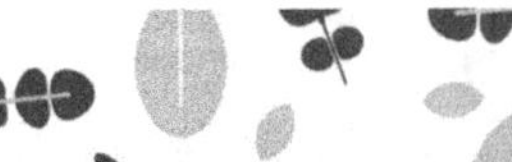
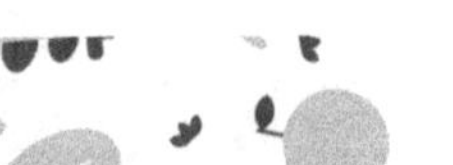
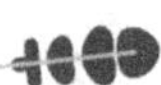

Preparation: 10'   **Cooking:** 20'   **Servings:** 4

ONION RINGS

INGREDIENTS

- 2 sweet onions, large
- .66 c. soy milk, unsweetened
- .66 c. flour
- 1 tbsp. nutritional yeast
- 1 tsp. garlic powder
- 1 tsp. paprika, smoked
- 1 tsp. sea salt
- 1 c. panko bread crumbs (vegan)

DIRECTIONS

1. Preheat the oven to 350°F before lining a large baking sheet with either non-stick silicone or kitchen parchment.
2. In a medium-sized bowl, whisk the flour, nutritional yeast, garlic powder, smoked paprika, sea salt, and unsweetened soy milk until no clumps remain. Set this batter aside while you prepare the onions.
3. Peel the large sweet onions and then cut them into rings about ¼ of 1-inch thick before carefully separating them from each other, avoiding breaking them.
4. Place the panko bread crumbs in a separate bowl for mixing and then begin to coat the onion rings. To do this, you first dip the rings 1–2 at a time in the batter. After the rings are coated in the batter, you then coat them in the panko bread crumb mixture.
5. Place the battered and coated onion rings on the prepared baking pans and allow them to cook for 20 minutes, flipping them over halfway through the cooking time to ensure they become evenly crispy.
6. Serve the onion rings immediately either on their own or with your favorite dipping sauce.

NUTRITION

Calories: 256.
Protein: 7 g.
Fat: 1 g.

Total carbohydrates: 49 g.
Net carbohydrates: 46 g.

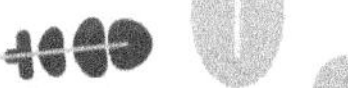
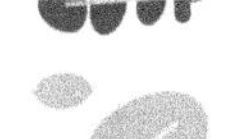
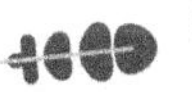

Preparation: 5'   Cooking: 0'   Servings: 1

CHOCOLATE PUDDING

INGREDIENTS

- 1 banana
- 2–4 tbsps. non-dairy milk
- 2 tbsps. unsweetened cocoa powder
- 2 tbsps. sugar (optional)
- ½ ripe avocado or 1 c. silken tofu (optional)

DIRECTIONS

1. In a small blender, add milk, cocoa powder, sugar (if using), and avocado (if using). Purée until smooth.
2. Alternatively, in a small bowl, mash the banana very well, and stir in the remaining ingredients.

NUTRITION

Calories: 244.
Protein: 4 g.
Total fat: 3 g.

Saturated fat: 1 g.
Carbohydrates: 59 g.
Fiber: 8 g.

Preparation: 10'   Cooking: 0'   Servings: 8

AVOCADO PUDDING

INGREDIENTS

- 2 ripe avocados, peeled, pitted, and cut into pieces
- 1 tbsp. fresh lime juice
- 14 oz. can coconut milk
- 80 drops of liquid Stevia
- 2 tsps. vanilla extract

DIRECTIONS

1. Add all ingredients into the blender and blend until smooth.
2. Serve and enjoy.

NUTRITION

Calories: 317.
Fat: 30.1 g.
Carbohydrates: 9.3 g.

Sugar: 0.4 g.
Protein: 3.4 g.
Cholesterol: 0 mg.

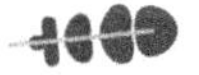

Preparation: 30'   **Cooking:** 20'   **Servings:** 4

ALMOND BUTTER BROWNIES

INGREDIENTS

- 1 scoop protein powder
- 2 tbsp. cocoa powder
- ½ c. almond butter, melted
- 1 c. bananas, overripe

DIRECTIONS

1. Take a waffle iron, oil generously, and preheat.
2. Take a large bowl and add the dry ingredients. Stir well together.
3. Put the wet ingredients into another bowl and stir until combined.
4. Stir the dry and wet together until combined.
5. Pour the mixture into the waffle iron and cook at medium temperature for 20 minutes.
6. Open carefully and remove.
7. Serve and enjoy.

NUTRITION

Calories: 132.
Fat: 5 g.

Carbohydrates: 14 g.
Protein: 3 g.

Preparation: 3 h 10'   **Cooking:** 0'   **Servings:** 2

RASPBERRY CHIA PUDDING

INGREDIENTS

- 4 tbsp. chia seeds
- 1 c. coconut milk
- ½ c. raspberries

DIRECTIONS

1. Add raspberry and coconut milk in a blender and blend until smooth.
2. Pour mixture into the mason jar.
3. Add chia seeds in a jar and stir well.
4. Close the jar tightly with the lid and shake well.
5. Place in refrigerator for 3 hours.
6. Serve chilled and enjoy.

NUTRITION

Calories: 361.
Fat: 33.4 g.
Carbohydrates: 13.3 g.

Sugar: 5.4 g.
Protein: 6.2 g.

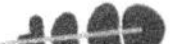

Preparation: 10'   **Cooking:** 0'   **Servings:** 12

CHOCOLATE FUDGE

INGREDIENTS

- 4 oz. unsweetened dark chocolate
- ¾ c. coconut butter
- 15 drops liquid Stevia
- 1 tsp. vanilla extract

DIRECTIONS

1. Melt coconut butter and dark chocolate.
2. Add ingredients to a large bowl and combine well.
3. Pour mixture into a silicone loaf pan and place it in refrigerator until set.
4. Cut into pieces and serve.

NUTRITION

Calories: 157.   Sugar: 1 g.
Fat: 14.1 g.   Protein: 2.3 g.
Carbohydrates: 6.1 g.   Cholesterol: 0 mg.

Preparation: 10'   **Cooking:** 0'   **Servings:** 8

CARROT ENERGY BALLS

INGREDIENTS

- 1 large carrot, grated
- 1 ½ c. old-fashioned oats
- 1 c. raisins
- 1 c. dates, pitied
- 1 c. coconut flakes
- ¼ tsp. ground cloves
- ½ tsp. ground cinnamon

DIRECTIONS

1. In your food processor, pulse all ingredients until it forms a sticky and uniform mixture.
2. Shape the batter into equal balls.
3. Place in your refrigerator until ready to serve. Bon appétit!

NUTRITION

Calories: 495.
Fat: 21.1 g.

Carbohydrates: 58.4 g.
Protein: 22.1 g.

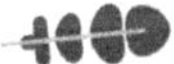
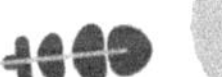

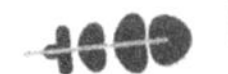

Preparation: 15'   **Cooking:** 10'   **Servings:** 4

CRUNCHY SWEET POTATO BITES

INGREDIENTS

- 4 sweet potatoes, peeled and grated
- 2 chia eggs
- ¼ c. nutritional yeast
- 2 tbsps. tahini
- 2 tbsps. chickpea flour
- 1 tsp. shallot powder
- 1 tsp. garlic powder
- 1 tsp. paprika
- Sea salt and ground black pepper, to taste

DIRECTIONS

1. Start by preheating your oven to 395°F. Line a baking pan with parchment paper or a Silpat mat.
2. Thoroughly combine all the ingredients until everything is well mixed.
3. Roll the batter into equal balls and place them in your refrigerator for about 1 hour.
4. Bake these balls for approximately 25 minutes, turning them over halfway through the cooking time. Bon appétit!

NUTRITION

Calories: 215.
Fat: 4.5 g.

Carbohydrates: 35 g.
Protein: 8.7 g.

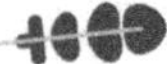

Preparation: 15'   Cooking: 10'   Servings: 4

ROASTED GLAZED BABY CARROTS

INGREDIENTS

- 2 lbs. baby carrots
- ¼ c. olive oil
- ¼ c. apple cider vinegar
- ½ tsp. red pepper flakes
- Sea salt and freshly ground black pepper, to taste
- 1 tbsp. agave syrup
- 2 tbsps. soy sauce
- 1 tbsp. fresh cilantro, minced

DIRECTIONS

1. Start by preheating your oven at 395°F.
2. Then, toss the carrots with olive oil, vinegar, red pepper, salt, black pepper, agave syrup, and soy sauce.
3. Roast the carrots for about 30 minutes, rotating the pan once or twice. Garnish with fresh cilantro and serve. Bon appétit!

NUTRITION

Calories: 165.
Fat: 10.1 g.

Carbohydrates: 16.5 g.
Protein: 1.4 g.

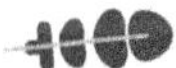
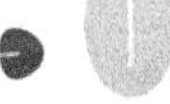
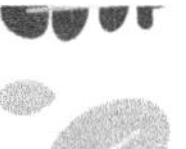
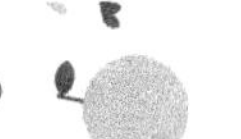
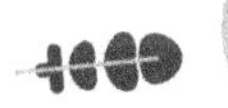

CHAPTER 11
Sauces, Dressings, and Dips

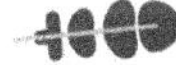

Preparation: 15'   Cooking: 15'   Servings: 6

WHITE BEANS DIP

INGREDIENTS

- ½ c. olive oil
- 2 tbsps. garlic cloves, chopped
- 2 (8 oz.) cans of white beans, drained and rinsed
- ¼ c. fresh lemon juice
- 4 tbsps. fresh parsley, chopped and divided
- 1 tsp. ground cumin
- ¼ tbsp. salt
- 1 tsp. ground white pepper

DIRECTIONS

1. In a small saucepan, place the olive oil and garlic over medium-low heat and cook for about 2 minutes, stirring continuously.
2. Remove the pan with garlic oil from heat and let it cool slightly.
3. Strain the garlic oil, reserving both the oil and garlic in separate bowls.
4. In a food processor, place the beans, garlic, lemon juice, 2 tbsps. of parsley, cumin, and pulse until smooth.
5. While the motor is running, add the reserved oil and pulse until light and smooth.
6. Transfer the dip into a bowl and stir in salt and white pepper.
7. Serve with the garnishing of remaining parsley.

NUTRITION

Calories: 263.
Total fat: 18.1 g.
Saturated fat: 2.5 g.
Cholesterol: 0 mg.
Sodium: 630 mg.

Total carbohydrates: 20.2 g.
Fiber: 5.7 g.
Sugar: 0.3 g.
Protein: 7 g.

Preparation: 15'　　　**Cooking:** 11'　　　**Servings:** 5

EDAMAME HUMMUS

INGREDIENTS

- 10 oz. frozen edamame pods
- 1 ripe avocado, peeled, pitted, and chopped roughly
- ½ c. fresh cilantro, chopped
- ¼ c. scallion, chopped
- 1 jalapeño pepper
- 1 garlic clove, peeled
- 2–3 tbsps. fresh lime juice
- Salt and ground black pepper, to taste
- ¼ c. avocado oil
- 2 tbsps. fresh basil leaves

DIRECTIONS

1. In a small pot of boiling water, cook the edamame pods for 6–8 minutes.
2. Drain the edamame pods and let them cool completely.
3. Remove soybeans from the pods.
4. In a food processor, add edamame and the remaining ingredients (except for oil) and pulse until mostly pureed.
5. While the motor is running, add the reserved oil and pulse until light and smooth.
6. Transfer the hummus into a bowl and serve with the garnishing of remaining basil leaves.

NUTRITION

Calories: 339.
Total fat: 33.8 g.
Saturated fat: 4.3 g.
Cholesterol: 0 mg.
Sodium: 27 mg.

Total carbohydrates: 6.3 g.
Fiber: 3.1 g.
Sugar: 0.3 g.
Protein: 5.1 g.

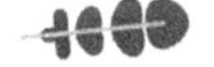

Preparation: 10' Cooking: 2' Servings: 4

BEANS MAYONNAISE

INGREDIENTS

- 1 (15 oz.) can white beans, drained and rinsed
- 2 tbsps. apple cider vinegar
- 1\tbsp. fresh lemon juice
- 2 tbsps. yellow mustard
- ¾ tsp. salt
- 2 garlic cloves, peeled
- 2 tbsps. aquafaba (liquid from the can of beans)

DIRECTIONS

1. In a food processor, add all ingredients (except for oil) and pulse until mostly pureed.
2. While the motor is running, add the reserved oil and pulse until light and smooth.
3. Transfer the mayonnaise into a container and refrigerate to chill before serving.

NUTRITION

Calories: 8.
Total fat: 1.1 g.
Saturated fat: 0.1 g.
Cholesterol: 0 mg.
Sodium: 559 mg.

Total carbohydrates: 14.3 g.
Fiber: 4.1 g.
Sugar: 0.2 g.
Protein: 5.2 g.

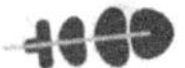

Preparation: 10'   **Cooking**: 0'   **Servings**: 5

CASHEW CREAM

INGREDIENTS

- 1 c. raw, unsalted cashews, soaked for 12 hours and drained
- ½ c. water
- 1 tbsp. nutritional yeast
- 1 tsp. fresh lemon juice
- ⅛ tsp. salt

DIRECTIONS

1. In a food processor, add all the ingredients and pulse at high speed until creamy and smooth.
2. Serve immediately.

NUTRITION

Calories: 165.
Total fat: 12.8 g.
Saturated fat: 2.5 g.
Cholesterol: 0 mg.
Sodium: 65 mg.

Total carbohydrates: 9.9 g.
Fiber: 1.3 g.
Sugar: 1.4 g.
Protein: 5.1 g.

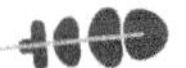

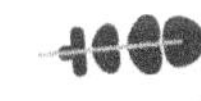

Preparation: 15'   **Cooking:** 0'   **Servings:** 4

LEMON TAHINI

INGREDIENTS

- ¼ c. fresh lemon juice
- 4 medium garlic cloves, pressed
- ½ c. tahini
- ½ tsp. fine sea salt
- Pinch of ground cumin
- 6 tbsps. ice water

DIRECTIONS

1. In a medium bowl, combine the lemon juice and garlic and set aside for 10 minutes.
2. Through a fine-mesh sieve, strain the mixture into another medium bowl, pressing the garlic solids.
3. Discard the garlic solids.
4. In the lemon juice bowl, add the tahini, salt, and cumin, and whisk until well blended.
5. Slowly, add water, 2 tbsps. at a time, whisking well after each addition.

NUTRITION

Calories: 187.
Total fat: 16.3 g.
Saturated fat: 2.4 g.
Cholesterol: 0 mg.
Sodium: 273 mg.

Total carbohydrates: 7.7 g.
Fiber: 2.9 g.
Sugar: 0.5 g.
Protein: 5.4 g

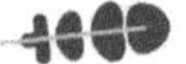

Preparation: 35' Cooking: 11' Servings: 12

KETO-VEGAN KETCHUP

INGREDIENTS

- ⅛ tsp. mustard powder
- ⅛ tsp. cloves, ground
- ¼ tsp. paprika
- ½ tsp. garlic powder
- ¾ tsp. onion powder
- 1 tsp. sea salt
- 3 tbsp. apple cider vinegar
- ¼ c. powdered monk fruit
- 1 c. water
- 6 oz. tomato paste

DIRECTIONS

1. In a little saucepan, whisk together all the ingredients.
2. Cover the pan and put it to low heat and simmer for 30 minutes, stirring occasionally.
3. Once reduced, add to the blender and puree until it has a smooth consistency.

NUTRITION

Calories: 13.
Carbohydrates: 2 g.

Protein: 0 g.
Fat: 0 g.

Preparation: 5'   **Cooking:** 5'   **Servings:** 6

AVOCADO HUMMUS

INGREDIENTS

- 1 tbsp. cilantro, finely chopped
- ⅛ tsp. cumin
- 1 clove garlic
- 3 tbsps. lime juice
- 1 ½ tbsps. Tahini
- 1 ½ tbsps. olive oil
- 2 avocados, medium cored and peeled
- 15 oz. chickpeas, drained
- Salt and pepper to taste

DIRECTIONS

1. In a food processor, add garlic, lime juice, tahini, olive oil, chickpeas, and pulse until combined.
2. Add cumin and avocados and blend until smooth consistency, approximately 2 minutes.
3. Add salt and pepper to taste.

NUTRITION

Calories: 310.
Carbohydrates: 26 g.

Protein: 8 g.
Fat: 20 g.

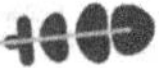

Preparation: 5'   **Cooking:** 5'   **Servings:** 6

GUACAMOLE

INGREDIENTS

- 3 tbsps. tomato, diced
- 3 tbsps. onion, diced
- 2 tbsps. cilantro, chopped
- 2 tbsps. jalapeño juice
- ¼ tsp. garlic powder
- ½ tsp. salt
- ½ lime, squeezed
- 2 big avocados
- 1 jalapeño, diced

DIRECTIONS

1. Using a molcajete, crush the diced jalapeños until soft.
2. Add the avocados to the molcajete.
3. Squeeze the lime juice from ½ of the lime on top of the avocados.
4. Add the jalapeño juice, garlic, and salt and mix until smooth.
5. Once smooth, add in the onion, cilantro, and tomato and stir to mix.

NUTRITION

Calories: 127.
Carbohydrates: 9.3 g.

Protein: 2.4 g.
Fat: 10.2 g.

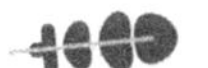

Preparation: 5'   Cooking:5'   Servings: 6

KETO-VEGAN MAYO

INGREDIENTS

- ½ c. extra virgin olive oil
- ½ c. almond milk, unsweetened
- ¼ tsp. xanthan gum
- Pinch of white pepper, ground
- Pinch of Himalayan salt
- 1 tsp. Dijon mustard
- 2 tsp. apple cider vinegar

DIRECTIONS

1. In a blender, place milk, pepper, salt, mustard, and vinegar.
2. Turn the blender to high speed and slowly add xanthan, then the olive oil.
3. Remove it from the blender and allow cooling for 2 hours in the refrigerator.
4. During cooling, the mixture will thicken.

NUTRITION

Calories: 160.4.   Protein: 0 g.
Carbohydrates: 0.2 g.   Fat: 18 g.

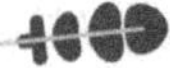

Preparation: 10'   **Cooking:** 10'   **Servings:** 4

PEANUT SAUCE

INGREDIENTS

- ½ tsp. Thai red curry paste
- 1 tsp. coconut oil
- 1 tsp. soy sauce
- 1 tsp. chili garlic sauce
- 1 tbsp. sweetener of your choice
- ⅓ c. coconut milk
- ¼ c. peanut butter, smooth

DIRECTIONS

1. Using a microwave-safe dish, add the peanut butter and heat for about 30 seconds.
2. Whisk into the peanut butter the soy sauce, sweetener, and chili garlic, then set to the side.
3. Warm a little saucepan over medium heat and add oil.
4. Cook the Thai red curry paste until fragrant, then add to a microwave-safe bowl.
5. Continuously stir the peanut mixture as you add the coconut milk. Stir until well-combined.
6. Enjoy at room temperature or warmed.

NUTRITION

Calories: 151.

Carbohydrates: 4 g.

Protein: 4 g.

Fat: 13 g.

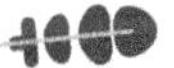
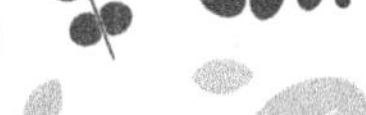
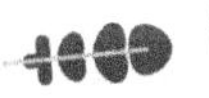

Preparation: 10'   **Cooking:** 10'   **Servings:** 8

PISTACHIO DIP

INGREDIENTS

- 2 tbsps. lemon juice
- 1 tsp. extra virgin olive oil
- 2 tbsps. tahini
- 2 tbsps. parsley, chopped
- 2 cloves of garlic
- ½ c. pistachios shelled
- 15 oz. garbanzo beans, save the liquid from the can
- Salt and pepper to taste

DIRECTIONS

1. Using a food processor, add pistachios, pepper, salt, lemon juice, olive oil, tahini, parsley, garlic, and garbanzo beans. Pulse until mixed.
2. Using the liquid from the garbanzo beans, add to the dip, while slowly blending, until it reaches the desired consistency.
3. Enjoy at room temperature or warmed.

NUTRITION

Calories: 88.   Protein: 2.5 g.
Carbohydrates: 9 g.   Fat: 3 g.

Preparation: 45'   Cooking: 45'   Servings: 1

SMOKEY TOMATO JAM

INGREDIENTS

- ½ tsp. white wine vinegar
- ½ tsp. salt
- ⅓ tsp. smoked paprika
- Pinch black pepper
- ¼ c. coconut sugar
- 2 lbs. tomatoes

DIRECTIONS

1. Over medium-high heat, bring a big pot of water to a boil.
2. Fill a big bowl with ice and water.
3. Carefully place the tomatoes into the boiling water for 1 minute and then remove, and immediately put into the ice water.
4. While tomatoes are in the ice water, peel them by hand and then transfer them to a clean cutting surface.
5. Empty the pot of water.
6. Chop the tomatoes and place back into the pot; add the coconut sugar and stir to combine.
7. Bring the pot back to medium heat and the tomatoes to a boil, cooking for 15 minutes.
8. Stir in the paprika, pepper, and salt, and then bring the temperature down to the lowest setting. Let it cook until it becomes thick, which is approximately 10 minutes.
9. Remove it from the heat while continuing to stir; add in white wine vinegar.

NUTRITION

Calories: 26.   Protein: 1.1 g.

Carbohydrates: 5.3 g.   Fat: 0.6 g

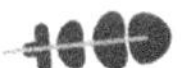

Preparation: 45' Cooking: 45' Servings: 16

TASTY RANCH DRESSING/DIP

INGREDIENTS

- ½ c. soy milk, unsweetened
- 1 tbsp. dill, chopped
- 2 tsp. parsley, chopped
- ¼ tsp. black pepper
- ½ tsp. onion powder
- ½ tsp. garlic powder
- 1 c. vegan mayonnaise

DIRECTIONS

1. In a medium bowl, whisk all the ingredients together until smooth. If dressing is too thick, add ¼ tbsp. of soy milk at a time until the desired consistency.
2. Transfer to an airtight container or jar and refrigerate for 1 hour.
3. Serve over leafy greens or as a dip.

NUTRITION

Calories: 93.
Carbohydrates: 0 g.

Protein: 0 g.
Fat: 9 g

Preparation: 20'   **Cooking**: 20'   **Servings**: 4

DOUBLE-BOILED COUNTRY STYLE FRIED POTATOES

INGREDIENTS

- 2 medium potatoes, cut into large chips
- ½ c. canola oil
- ¼ tsp. ground cumin
- ¼ tsp. paprika
- ¼ tsp. white pepper
- 3 tbsp. ketchup

DIRECTIONS

1. Soak or double boil the potatoes if you are on a low-potassium diet.
2. Heat oil in a skillet over medium heat.
3. Fry the potatoes for around 10 minutes until golden brown.
4. Drain potatoes, then sprinkle with cumin, pepper, and paprika.
5. Serve with ketchup or mayo.

NUTRITION

Calories: 156.
Fat: 0.1 g.
Carbohydrates: 21 g.
Protein: 2 g.

Sodium: 3 mg.
Potassium: 296 mg.
Phosphorous: 34 mg.

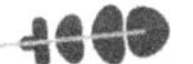

Preparation: 15'   Cooking: 20'   Servings: 4

BROCCOLI-ONION LATKES

INGREDIENTS

- 3 c. broccoli florets, diced
- ½ c. onion, chopped
- 2 large eggs, beaten
- 2 tbsp. all-purpose white flour
- 2 tbsp. olive oil

DIRECTIONS

1. Cook the broccoli for around 5 minutes until tender. Drain.
2. Mix the flour into the eggs.
3. Combine the onion, broccoli, and egg mixture and stir through.
4. Heat olive oil in a skillet on Medium-high.
5. Drop a spoon of the mixture onto the pan to make 4 latkes.
6. Cook each side until golden brown.
7. Drain on a paper towel and serve.

NUTRITION

Calories: 140.
Carbohydrates: 7 g.
Protein: 6 g.
Sodium: 58 mg.

Potassium: 276 mg.
Fats: 0.2 g.
Phosphorous: 101 mg.

CHAPTER 12
Vegetable Recipes

Preparation: 15'   **Cooking:** 30'   **Servings:** 4

CAULIFLOWER LATKE

INGREDIENTS

- 12 oz. cauliflower rice, cooked
- 1 egg, beaten
- ⅓ c. cornstarch
- Salt and pepper to taste
- ¼ c. vegetable oil, divided
- Chopped onion chives

DIRECTIONS

1. Squeeze excess water from the cauliflower rice using paper towels.
2. Place the cauliflower rice in a bowl.
3. Stir in the egg and cornstarch.
4. Season with salt and pepper.
5. Fill 2 tbsps. of oil into a pan over medium heat.
6. Add 2–3 tbsps. of the cauliflower mixture into the pan.
7. Cook for 3 minutes on each side.
8. Repeat until you've used up the rest of the batter.
9. Garnish with chopped chives.

NUTRITION

Calories: 209.   Protein: 3.4 g.
Fiber: 1.9 g.

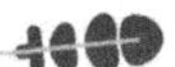

Preparation: 30' **Cooking:** 20' **Servings:** 4

ROASTED BRUSSELS SPROUTS

INGREDIENTS

- 1 lb. Brussels sprouts, sliced in half
- 1 tbsp. olive oil
- Salt and pepper to taste
- 2 tsps. balsamic vinegar
- ¼ c. pomegranate seeds
- ¼ c. goat cheese, crumbled

DIRECTIONS

1. Preheat your oven to 400°F.
2. Coat the Brussels sprouts with oil.
3. Sprinkle with salt and pepper.
4. Transfer to a baking pan.
5. Roast in the oven for 20 minutes.
6. Drizzle with the vinegar.
7. Sprinkle with the seeds and cheese before serving.

NUTRITION

Calories: 117.
Fiber: 4.8 g.

Protein: 5.8 g.

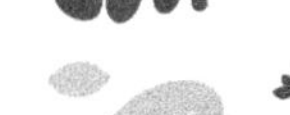
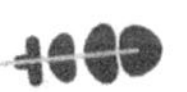

Preparation: 10'   Cooking: 0'   Servings: 6

BRUSSELS SPROUTS AND CRANBERRIES

INGREDIENTS

- 3 tbsps. lemon juice
- ¼ c. olive oil
- Salt and pepper to taste
- 1 lb. Brussels sprouts, sliced thinly
- ¼ c. dried cranberries, chopped
- ½ c. pecans, toasted and chopped
- ½ c. Parmesan cheese, shaved

DIRECTIONS

1. Mix the lemon juice, olive oil, salt, and pepper in a bowl.
2. Toss the Brussels sprouts, cranberries, and pecans in this mixture.
3. Sprinkle the Parmesan cheese on top.

NUTRITION

Calories: 245.   Fiber: 5 g.
Protein: 6.4 g.

Preparation: 15' **Cooking:** 10' **Servings:** 6

POTATO LATKE

INGREDIENTS

- 3 eggs, beaten
- 1 onion, grated
- 1 ½ tsps. baking powder
- Salt and pepper to taste
- 2 lbs. potatoes, peeled and grated
- ¼ c. all-purpose flour
- 4 tbsps. vegetable oil
- Chopped onion chives

DIRECTIONS

1. Prep your oven to 400°F.
2. Scourge eggs, onion, baking powder, salt, and pepper.
3. Squeeze moisture from the shredded potatoes using a paper towel.
4. Add potatoes to the egg mixture.
5. Stir in the flour.
6. Heat the oil into a pan over Medium setting.
7. Cook a small amount of the batter for 3–4 minutes per side.
8. Repeat. Garnish with the chives.

NUTRITION

Calories: 266.
Carbohydrates: 34.6 g.

Protein: 7.6 g.

Preparation: 15'   **Cooking:** 15'   **Servings:** 8

BROCCOLI RABE

INGREDIENTS

- 2 oranges, sliced in half
- 1 lb. broccoli rabe
- 2 tbsps. sesame oil, toasted
- Salt and pepper to taste
- 1 tbsp. sesame seeds, toasted

DIRECTIONS

1. Heat the oil into a pan over medium setting.
2. Add the oranges and cook until caramelized.
3. Transfer to a plate.
4. Put the broccoli in the pan and cook for 8 minutes.
5. Squeeze the oranges to release juice in a bowl.
6. Stir in the oil, salt, and pepper.
7. Coat the broccoli rabe with the mixture.
8. Sprinkle seeds on top.

NUTRITION

Calories: 59.   Protein: 2.2 g.
Carbohydrates: 4.1 g.

Preparation: 20'   **Cooking:** 35'   **Servings:** 10

WHIPPED POTATOES

INGREDIENTS

- 4 c. water
- 3 lb. potatoes, sliced into cubes
- 3 garlic cloves, crushed
- 6 tbsps. butter
- 10 sage leaves
- ½ c. Greek yogurt
- ¼ c. low-fat milk
- Bay leaves

DIRECTIONS

1. Cook potatoes in water for 30 minutes.
2. Drain.
3. Cook garlic in butter for 1 minute over medium heat.
4. Add the sage and bay leaves and cook for 5 more minutes.
5. Discard the garlic and bay leaves.
6. Use a fork to mash the potatoes.
7. Whip using an electric mixer while gradually adding the butter, yogurt, and milk.
8. Season with salt.

NUTRITION

Calories: 169.   Protein: 4.2 g.
Carbohydrates: 22 g.

Preparation: 15'   **Cooking**: 4'   **Servings**: 4

QUINOA AVOCADO SALAD

INGREDIENTS

- 2 tbsps. balsamic vinegar
- ¼ c. cream
- ¼ c. buttermilk
- 5 tbsps. lemon juice
- 1 clove garlic, grated
- 2 tbsps. shallot, minced
- Salt and pepper to taste
- 2 tbsps. avocado oil, divided
- 1 ¼ c. quinoa, cooked
- 2 heads endive, sliced
- 2 firm pears, sliced thinly
- 2 avocados, sliced
- ¼ c. fresh dill, chopped

DIRECTIONS

1. Combine the vinegar, cream, milk, 1 tbsp. lemon juice, garlic, shallot, salt, and pepper in a bowl.
2. Pour 1 tbsp. oil into a pan over medium heat.
3. Heat the quinoa for 4 minutes.
4. Transfer quinoa to a plate.
5. Toss the endive and pears in a mixture of remaining oil, remaining lemon juice, salt, and pepper.
6. Transfer to a plate.
7. Toss the avocado in the reserved dressing.
8. Add to the plate.
9. Top with the dill and quinoa.

NUTRITION

Calories: 431.   Protein: 6.6 g.
Fiber: 6 g.

Preparation: 20'   Cooking: 20'   Servings: 4

ROASTED SWEET POTATOES

INGREDIENTS

- 2 potatoes, sliced into wedges
- 2 tbsps. olive oil, divided
- Salt and pepper to taste
- 1 red bell pepper, chopped
- ¼ c. fresh cilantro, chopped
- 1 garlic, minced
- 2 tbsps. almonds, toasted and sliced
- 1 tbsp. lime juice

DIRECTIONS

1. Preheat your oven to 425°F.
2. Toss the sweet potatoes in oil and salt.
3. Transfer to a baking pan.
4. Roast for 20 minutes.
5. In a bowl, combine the red bell pepper, cilantro, garlic, and almonds.
6. In another bowl, mix the lime juice, remaining oil, salt, and pepper.
7. Drizzle this mixture over the red bell pepper mixture.
8. Serve sweet potatoes with the red bell pepper mixture.

NUTRITION

Calories: 146.
Fiber: 2.9 g.

Protein: 2.3 g.

Preparation: 20'   **Cooking:** 15'   **Servings:** 4

CAULIFLOWER SALAD

INGREDIENTS

- 8 c. cauliflower florets
- 5 tbsps. olive oil, divided
- Salt and pepper to taste
- 1 c. parsley
- 1 garlic clove, minced
- 2 tbsps. lemon juice
- ¼ c. almonds, toasted and sliced
- 3 c. arugula
- 2 tbsps. olives, sliced
- ¼ c. feta, crumbled

DIRECTIONS

1. Preheat your oven to 425°F.
2. Toss the cauliflower in a mixture of 1 tbsp. olive oil, salt, and pepper.
3. Place in a baking pan and roast for 15 minutes.
4. Put the parsley, remaining oil, garlic, lemon juice, salt, and pepper in a blender.
5. Pulse until smooth.
6. Place the roasted cauliflower in a salad bowl.
7. Stir in the rest of the ingredients along with the parsley dressing.

NUTRITION

Calories: 198.   Protein: 5.4 g.
Fiber: 4.1 g.

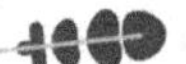

Preparation: 20'   **Cooking:** 30'   **Servings:** 8

GARLIC MASHED POTATOES AND TURNIPS

INGREDIENTS

- 1 head garlic
- 1 tsp. olive oil
- 1 lb. turnips, sliced into cubes
- 2 lbs. potatoes, sliced into cubes
- ½ c. almond milk
- ½ c. Parmesan cheese, grated
- 1 tbsp. fresh thyme, chopped
- 1 tbsp. fresh chives, chopped
- 2 tbsps. butter

DIRECTIONS

1. Preheat your oven to 375°F.
2. Slice the tip off the garlic head.
3. Dash little oil and roast in the oven for 45 minutes.
4. Boil the turnips and potatoes in a pot with water for 30 minutes or until tender.
5. Add all the ingredients into a food processor along with the garlic.
6. Pulse until smooth.

NUTRITION

Calories: 141.   Protein: 4.6 g.
Fiber: 3.1 g.

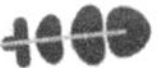
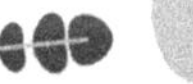
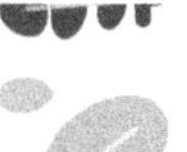
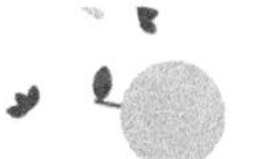
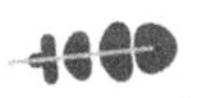

Preparation: 15'   **Cooking:** 20'   **Servings:** 8

GREEN BEANS

INGREDIENTS

- 1 shallot, chopped
- 24 oz. green beans
- Salt and pepper to taste
- ½ tsp. smoked paprika
- 1 tsp. lemon juice
- 2 tsps. vinegar

DIRECTIONS

1. Preheat your oven to 450°F.
2. Stir in the shallot and beans.
3. Season with salt, pepper, and paprika.
4. Roast for 10 minutes.
5. Drizzle with lemon juice and vinegar.
6. Roast for another 2 minutes.

NUTRITION

Calories: 49.   Protein: 2.9 g.
Fiber: 3 g.

Preparation: 15' Cooking: 10' Servings: 4

COCONUT BRUSSELS SPROUTS

INGREDIENTS

- 1 lb. Brussels sprouts, trimmed and sliced in half
- 2 tbsps. coconut oil
- ¼ c. coconut water
- 1 tbsp. soy sauce

DIRECTIONS

1. In a skillet over medium heat, stir the coconut oil and cook the Brussels sprouts for 4 minutes.
2. Pour in the coconut water.
3. Cook for 3 minutes.
4. Add the soy sauce and cook for another 1 minute.

NUTRITION

Calories: 114. Protein: 4 g.
Fiber: 4.3 g.

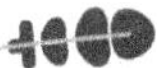
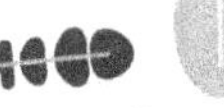
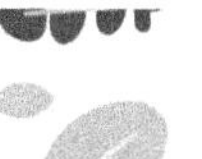

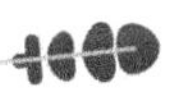

Preparation: 5' Cooking: 45' Servings: 8

CREAMY POLENTA

INGREDIENTS

- 1 ⅓ c. cornmeal
- 6 c. water
- Salt to taste

DIRECTIONS

1. Add all the ingredients in a pan over medium-high heat.
2. Boil and then simmer for 5 minutes.
3. Reduce the heat to low.
4. Stir until creamy for 45 minutes.
5. Let it sit before serving.

NUTRITION

Calories: 74.
Fiber: 3 g.

Protein: 1.6 g.

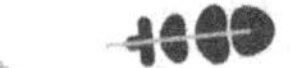

Preparation: 20'   **Cooking:** 25'   **Servings:** 4

SKILLET QUINOA

INGREDIENTS

- 1 c. sweet potato, cubed
- ½ c. water
- 1 tbsp. olive oil
- 1 onion, chopped
- 3 cloves garlic, minced
- 1 tsp. ground cumin
- 1 tsp. ground coriander
- ½ tsp. chili powder
- ½ tsp. dried oregano
- 15 oz. black beans, rinsed
- and drained
- 15 oz. roasted tomatoes
- 1 ¼ c. vegetable broth
- 1 c. frozen corn
- 1 c. quinoa (uncooked)
- Salt to taste
- ½ c. light sour cream
- ½ c. fresh cilantro leaves

DIRECTIONS

1. Add the water and sweet potato to a pan over medium heat.
2. Bring to a boil.
3. Decrease heat and cook sweet potatoes.
4. Add the oil and onion.
5. Cook for 3 minutes.
6. Cook garlic and spices for 1 minute.
7. Add the rest of the ingredients, except the sour cream and cilantro.
8. Cook for 20 minutes.
9. Serve with sour cream and top with the cilantro before serving.

NUTRITION

Calories: 421.   Protein: 16 g.
Fiber: 11 g.

Preparation: 10'   Cooking: 15'   Servings: 6

GREEN BEANS WITH BALSAMIC SAUCE

INGREDIENTS

- 2 shallots, sliced
- 8 c. green beans, trimmed
- 2 tbsps. olive oil
- Salt and pepper to taste
- 2 tbsps. balsamic vinegar
- ¼ c. Parmesan cheese, grated

DIRECTIONS

1. Preheat your oven to 425°F.
2. Line your baking with foil.
3. In the pan, toss the shallots and beans in oil, salt, and pepper.
4. Roast in the oven for 15 minutes.
5. Drizzle with the vinegar and top with cheese.

NUTRITION

Calories: 78.   Protein: 1.9 g.
Fiber: 0.6 g.

CHAPTER 13

Desserts

Preparation: 20'   Cooking: 25'   Servings: 6

APPLE CRUMBLE

INGREDIENTS

For the filling:
- 4–5 apples, cored and chopped (about 6 c.)
- ½ c. unsweetened applesauce or ¼ c. water
- 2–3 tbsps. unrefined sugar (coconut, date, Sucanat, or maple syrup)
- 1 tsp. ground cinnamon
- Pinch sea salt

For the crumble:
- 2 tbsps. almond butter, or cashew or sunflower seed butter
- 2 tbsps. maple syrup
- 1 ½ c. rolled oats
- ½ c. walnuts, finely chopped
- ½ tsp. ground cinnamon
- 2–3 tbsps. unrefined granular sugar (coconut, date, Sucanat)

DIRECTIONS

1. Prepare the ingredients.
2. Preheat the oven to 350°F. Put the apples and applesauce in an 8-inch-square baking dish, and sprinkle with sugar, cinnamon, and salt. Toss to combine.
3. In a medium bowl, mix the almond butter and maple syrup until smooth and creamy. Add the oats, walnuts, cinnamon, and sugar and stir to coat, using your hands if necessary. (If you have a small food processor, pulse the oats and walnuts together before adding them to the mix.)
4. Sprinkle the topping over the apples, and put the dish in the oven.
5. Bake for 20–25 minutes, or until the fruit is soft and the topping is lightly browned.

NUTRITION

Calories: 195.
Fat: 7 g.
Carbohydrates: 6 g.

Sugar: 2 g.
Protein: 24 g.
Cholesterol: 65 mg.

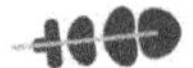

Preparation: 15'   **Cooking:** 0'   **Servings:** 12

CASHEW-CHOCOLATE TRUFFLES

INGREDIENTS

- 1 c. raw cashews, soaked in water overnight
- ¾ c. pitted dates
- 2 tbsps. coconut oil
- 1 c. unsweetened shredded coconut, divided
- 1–2 tbsps. cocoa powder, to taste

DIRECTIONS

1. Prepare the ingredients.
2. In a food processor, combine the cashews, dates, coconut oil, ½ c. of shredded coconut, and cocoa powder. Pulse until fully mixed; it will resemble chunky cookie dough. Spread the remaining ½ c. of shredded coconut on a plate.
3. Form the mixture into tablespoon-size balls and roll on the plate to cover with the shredded coconut. Transfer to a parchment paper-lined plate or baking sheet. Repeat to make 12 truffles.
4. Place the truffles in the refrigerator for 1 hour to set. Transfer the truffles to a storage container or freezer-safe bag and seal.

NUTRITION

Calories: 160.
Fat: 1 g.
Carbohydrates: 1 g.

Sugar: 0.5 g.
Protein: 22 g.
Cholesterol: 60 mg.

Preparation: 20'   Cooking: 20'   Servings: 1

BANANA CHOCOLATE CUPCAKES

INGREDIENTS

- 3 medium bananas
- 1 c. non-dairy milk
- 2 tbsps. almond butter
- 1 tsp. apple cider vinegar
- 1 tsp. pure vanilla extract
- 1¼ c. whole grain flour
- ½ c. rolled oats
- ¼ c. coconut sugar (optional)
- 1 tsp. baking powder
- ½ tsp. baking soda
- ½ c. unsweetened cocoa powder
- ¼ c. chia seeds, or sesame seeds
- Pinch sea salt
- ¼ c. dark chocolate chips, dried cranberries, or raisins (optional)

DIRECTIONS

1. Prepare the ingredients.
2. Preheat the oven to 350°F. Lightly grease the c. of 2 6-cup muffin tins or line with paper muffin cups.
3. Put the bananas, milk, almond butter, vinegar, and vanilla in a blender and purée until smooth. Or stir together in a large bowl until smooth and creamy.
4. Put the flour, oats, sugar (if using), baking powder, baking soda, cocoa powder, chia seeds, salt, and chocolate chips in another large bowl, and stir to combine. Mix the wet and dry ingredients, stirring as little as possible. Spoon into muffin cups, and bake for 20–25 minutes. Take the cupcakes out of the oven and let them cool fully before taking them out of the muffin tins since they'll be very moist.

NUTRITION

Calories: 295.
Fat: 17 g.
Carbohydrates: 4 g.

Sugar: 0.1 g.
Protein: 29 g.
Cholesterol: 260 mg.

Preparation: 15'　　　　**Cooking:** 5'　　　　**Servings:** 4

MINTY FRUIT SALAD

INGREDIENTS

- ¼ c. lemon juice (about 2 small lemons)
- 4 tsps. maple syrup or agave syrup
- 2 c. chopped pineapple
- 2 c. chopped strawberries
- 2 c. raspberries
- 1 c. blueberries
- 8 fresh mint leaves

DIRECTIONS

1. Prepare the ingredients.
2. Beginning with 1 mason jar, add the ingredients in this order:
3. 1 tbsp. of lemon juice, 1 tsp. of maple syrup, ½ c. of pineapple, ½ c. of strawberries, ½ c. of raspberries, ¼ c. of blueberries, and 2 mint leaves.
4. Repeat to fill 3 more jars. Close the jars tightly with lids.
5. Place the airtight jars in the refrigerator for up to 3 days.

NUTRITION

Calories: 339.
Fat: 17.5 g.
Carbohydrates: 2 g.

Sugar: 2 g.
Protein: 44 g.
Cholesterol: 100 mg.

Preparation: 20'   Cooking: 30'   Servings: 8

MANGO COCONUT CREAM PIE

INGREDIENTS

For the crust:
- ½ c. rolled oats
- 1 c. cashews
- 1 c. soft pitted dates

For the filling:
- 1 c. canned coconut milk
- ½ c. water
- 2 large mangos, peeled and chopped, or about 2 c. frozen chunks
- ½ c. unsweetened shredded coconut

DIRECTIONS

1. Prepare the ingredients.
2. Put all the crust ingredients in a food processor and pulse until it holds together. If you do not have a food processor, chop everything as finely as possible and use ½ c. cashew or almond butter in place of half the cashews. Press the mixture down firmly into an 8-inch pie or springform pan.
3. Put all the filling ingredients in a blender and purée until smooth (about 1 minute). It should be very thick, so you may have to stop and stir until it's smooth.
4. Pour the filling into the crust, use a rubber spatula to smooth the top, and put the pie in the freezer until set, about 30 minutes. Once frozen, it should be set out for about 15 minutes to soften before serving.
5. Top with a batch of Coconut Whipped Cream scooped on top of the pie once it's set. Finish it off with a sprinkling of toasted shredded coconut.

NUTRITION

Calories: 545.
Fat: 39.6 g.
Carbohydrates: 9.5 g.

Sugar: 3.1 g.
Protein: 43 g.
Cholesterol: 110 mg.

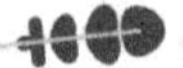
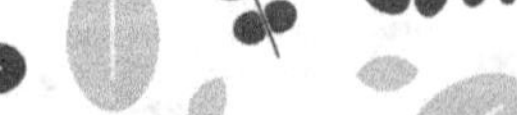
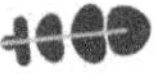

Preparation: 5' **Cooking:** 30' **Servings:** 4-6

CHERRY-VANILLA RICE PUDDING (PRESSURE COOKER)

INGREDIENTS

- 1 c. short-grain brown rice
- 1 ¾ c. non-dairy milk, plus more as needed
- 1 ½ c. water
- 4 tbsps. unrefined sugar or pure maple syrup (use 2 tbsps. if you use sweetened milk), plus more as needed
- 1 tsp. vanilla extract (use ½ tsp. if you use vanilla milk)
- Pinch salt
- ¼ c. dried cherries or ½ c. fresh or frozen pitted cherries

DIRECTIONS

1. Prepare the ingredients. In your electric pressure cooker's cooking pot, combine the rice, milk, water, sugar, vanilla, and salt.
2. Close and lock the lid, and select "High Pressure" for 30 minutes.
3. Once the time of cooking is completed, let the pressure release naturally, about 20 minutes. Unlock and remove the lid. Stir in the cherries and put the lid back on loosely for about 10 minutes.
4. Serve, adding more milk or sugar, as desired.

NUTRITION

Calories: 420.
Fat: 27.4 g.
Carbohydrates: 2 g.

Sugar: 0.3 g.
Protein: 46.3 g.
Cholesterol: 98 mg.

Preparation: 10'   Cooking: 20'   Servings: 4

LIME IN THE COCONUT CHIA PUDDING

INGREDIENTS

- Zest and juice of 1 lime
- 1 (14 oz.) can coconut milk
- 1–2 dates, or 1 tbsp. coconut or other unrefined sugar, or 1 tbsp. maple syrup, or 10–15 drops of pure liquid Stevia
- 2 tbsps. chia seeds, whole or ground
- 2 tsps. matcha green tea powder (optional)

DIRECTIONS

1. Prepare the ingredients.
2. Blend all the ingredients in a blender until smooth. Chill in the fridge for about 20 minutes, then serve topped with one or more of the topping ideas.
3. Try blueberries, blackberries, sliced strawberries, Coconut Whipped Cream, or toasted unsweetened coconut.

NUTRITION

Calories: 381.
Fat: 17.1 g.
Carbohydrates: 4.1 g.

Sugar: 0.6 g.
Protein: 50.6 g.
Cholesterol: 358 mg.

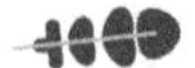
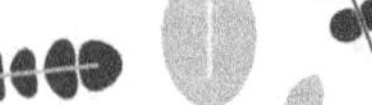

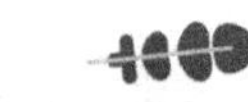

Preparation: 5' Cooking: 0' Servings: 1

MINT CHOCOLATE CHIP SORBET

INGREDIENTS

- 1 frozen banana
- 1 tbsp. almond butter, or peanut butter, or other nut or seed butter
- 2 tbsps. fresh mint, minced
- ¼ c. or less non-dairy milk (only if needed)
- 2–3 tbsps. non-dairy chocolate chips, or cocoa nibs
- 2–3 tbsps. goji berries (optional)

DIRECTIONS

1. Prepare the ingredients.
2. Put the banana, almond butter, and mint in a food processor or blender and purée until smooth.
3. Add the non-dairy milk if needed to keep blending (but only if needed, as this will make the texture less solid). Pulse the chocolate chips and goji berries (if using) into the mix so they're roughly chopped up.

NUTRITION

Calories: 299.
Fat: 16 g.
Carbohydrates: 3 g.

Sugar: 6 g.
Protein: 38 g.
Cholesterol: 108 mg.

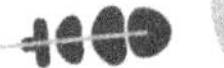

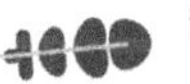

Preparation: 10' **Cooking:** 6' **Servings:** 4-6

PEACH-MANGO CRUMBLE (PRESSURE COOKER)

INGREDIENTS

- 3 c. chopped fresh or frozen peaches
- 3 c. chopped fresh or frozen mangos
- 4 tbsps. unrefined sugar or pure maple syrup, divided
- 1 c. gluten-free rolled oats
- ½ c. shredded coconut, sweetened or unsweetened
- 2 tbsps. coconut oil or vegan margarine

DIRECTIONS

1. Prepare the ingredients. In a 6–7-inch round baking dish, toss together the peaches, mangos, and 2 tbsps. of sugar. In a food processor, combine the oats, coconut, coconut oil, and remaining 2 tbsps. of sugar. Pulse until mixed. (If you use maple syrup, you'll need less coconut oil. Start with just the syrup and add oil if the mixture isn't sticking together.) Sprinkle the oat mixture over the fruit mixture.
2. Cover the dish with aluminum foil. Put a trivet in the bottom of your electric pressure cooker's cooking pot and pour in 1–2 c. of water. Using a foil sling or silicone helper handles, lower the pan onto the trivet.
3. Close and lock the lid, and select "High Pressure" for 6 minutes.
4. Once the time of cooking is completed, quickly release the pressure. Unlock and remove the lid.
5. Let it cool for a few minutes before carefully lifting out the dish with oven mitts or tongs. Scoop out portions to serve.

NUTRITION

Calories: 275.
Fat: 19 g.
Carbohydrates: 19 g.

Sugar: 4 g.
Protein: 14 g.
Cholesterol: 60 mg.

Preparation: 10' Cooking: 15' Servings: 12

ZESTY ORANGE-CRANBERRY ENERGY BITES

INGREDIENTS

- 2 tbsps. almond butter, or cashew or sunflower seed butter
- 2 tbsps. maple syrup, or brown rice syrup
- ¾ c. cooked quinoa
- ¼ c. sesame seeds, toasted
- 1 tbsp. chia seeds
- ½ tsp. almond extract, or vanilla extract
- Zest of 1 orange
- 1 tbsp. dried cranberries
- ¼ c. ground almonds

DIRECTIONS

1. Prepare the ingredients.
2. In a medium bowl, mix the almond or seed butter and syrup until smooth and creamy. Stir in the rest of the ingredients, and mix to ensure the consistency is holding together in a ball. Form the mix into 12 balls.
3. Place them on a baking sheet lined with parchment or waxed paper and put them in the fridge to set for about 15 minutes.
4. If your balls aren't holding together, it's likely because of the moisture content of your cooked quinoa. Add more almond or seed butter mixed with syrup until it all sticks together.

NUTRITION

Calories: 493.
Fat: 33 g.
Carbohydrates: 8 g.

Sugar: 9 g.
Protein: 47 g.
Cholesterol: 135 mg.

Preparation: 5' Cooking: 15' Servings: 24

ALMOND-DATE ENERGY BITES

INGREDIENTS

- 1 c. dates, pitted
- 1 c. unsweetened shredded coconut
- ¼ c. chia seeds
- ¾ c. ground almonds
- ¼ c. cocoa nibs, or non-dairy chocolate chips

DIRECTIONS

1. Purée everything in a food processor until crumbly and sticking together, pushing down the sides whenever necessary to keep it blending. If you do not have a food processor, you can mash soft Medjool dates. But if you're using harder baking dates, you'll have to soak them and then try to purée them in a blender.
2. Form the mix into 24 balls and place them on a baking sheet lined with parchment or waxed paper. Put in the fridge to set for about 15 minutes. Use the softest dates you can find. Medjool dates are the best for this purpose. The hard dates you see in the baking aisle of your supermarket will take a long time to blend up. If you use those, try soaking them in water for at least 1 hour before you start, and then drain them.

NUTRITION

Calories: 171.
Fat: 4 g.
Carbohydrates: 7 g.

Sugar: 7 g.
Protein: 22 g.
Cholesterol: 65 mg.

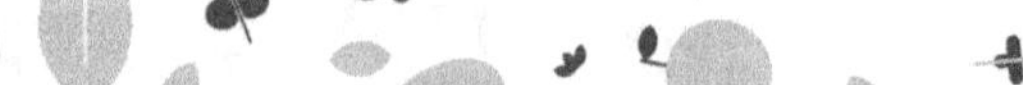

Preparation: 5'   Cooking: 6'   Servings: 4-6

PUMPKIN PIE CUPS (PRESSURE COOKER)

INGREDIENTS

- 1 c. canned pumpkin purée
- 1 c. non-dairy milk
- 6 tbsps. unrefined sugar or pure maple syrup (less if using sweetened milk), plus more for sprinkling
- ¼ c. spelt flour or whole grain flour
- ½ tsp. pumpkin pie spice
- Pinch salt

DIRECTIONS

1. Prepare the ingredients. In a medium bowl, stir together the pumpkin, milk, sugar, flour, pumpkin pie spice, and salt. Pour the mixture into 4 heatproof ramekins. Sprinkle a bit more sugar on the top of each, if you like. Put a trivet in the bottom of your electric pressure cooker's cooking pot and pour in 1–2 c. of water. Place the ramekins onto the trivet, stacking them if needed (3 on the bottom, 1 on top).
2. Close and lock the lid, and select "High Pressure" for 6 minutes.
3. Once the time of cooking is completed, quickly release the pressure. Unlock and remove the lid. Let it cool for a few minutes before carefully lifting out the ramekins with oven mitts or tongs. Let it cool for at least 10 minutes before serving.

NUTRITION

Calories: 152.
Fat: 4 g.
Carbohydrates: 4 g.

Sugar: 8 g.
Protein: 18 g.
Cholesterol: 51 mg.

Preparation: 15'   **Cooking:** 0'   **Servings:** 8

COCONUT AND ALMOND TRUFFLES

INGREDIENTS

- 1 c. pitted dates
- 1 c. almonds
- ½ c. sweetened cocoa powder, plus extra for coating
- ½ c. unsweetened shredded coconut
- ¼ c. pure maple syrup
- 1 tsp. vanilla extract
- 1 tsp. almond extract
- ¼ tsp. sea salt

DIRECTIONS

1. Prepare the ingredients.
2. In the bowl of a food processor, combine all the ingredients and process until smooth. Chill the mixture for about 1 hour.
3. Roll the mixture into balls and then roll the balls in cocoa powder to coat.
4. Serve immediately or keep chilled until ready to serve.

NUTRITION

Calories: 126.
Fat: 5 g.
Carbohydrates: 13 g.

Sugar: 7 g.
Protein: 5 g.
Cholesterol: 0 mg.

Preparation: 10'   Cooking: 5'   Servings: 4-6

FUDGY BROWNIES (PRESSURE COOKER)

INGREDIENTS

- 3 oz. dairy-free dark chocolate
- 1 tbsp. coconut oil or vegan margarine
- ½ c. applesauce
- 2 tbsps. unrefined sugar
- ⅓ c. whole grain flour
- ½ tsp. baking powder
- Pinch salt

DIRECTIONS

1. Prepare the ingredients. Put a trivet in your electric pressure cooker's cooking pot and pour in a 1–2 c. of water. Select "Sauté" or "Simmer." In a large heat-proof glass or ceramic bowl, combine the chocolate and coconut oil. Place the bowl over the top of your pressure cooker, as you would a double boiler. Stir occasionally until the chocolate is melted, then turn off the pressure cooker. Stir the applesauce and sugar into the chocolate mixture. Add the flour, baking powder, and salt and stir just until combined. Pour the batter into 3 heatproof ramekins. Put them in a heat-proof dish and cover with aluminum foil. Using a foil sling or silicone helper handles, lower the dish onto the trivet. (Alternately, cover each ramekin with foil and place them directly on the trivet, without the dish.)
2. Close and lock the lid, and select "High Pressure" for 5 minutes.
3. Once the time of cooking is completed, quickly release the pressure. Unlock and remove the lid.
4. Let it cool for a few minutes before carefully lifting out the dish, or ramekins, with oven mitts or tongs. Let it cool for a few minutes more before serving.
5. Top with fresh raspberries and an extra drizzle of melted chocolate.

NUTRITION

Calories: 256.
Fat: 29 g.
Carbohydrates: 1 g.

Sugar: 0.5 g.
Protein: 11 g.
Cholesterol: 84 mg.

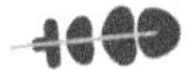

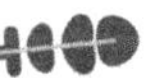

Preparation: 10'   **Cooking:** 15'   **Servings:** 8

CHOCOLATE MACAROONS

INGREDIENTS

- 1 c. unsweetened shredded coconut
- 2 tbsps. cocoa powder
- ⅔ c. coconut milk
- ¼ c. agave
- Pinch of sea salt

DIRECTIONS

1. Prepare the ingredients.
2. Preheat the oven to 350°F. Line a baking sheet with parchment paper. In a medium saucepan, cook all the ingredients over medium-high heat until a firm dough is formed. Scoop the dough into balls and place on the baking sheet.
3. Bake for 15 minutes, remove from the oven and let them cool on the baking sheet.
4. Serve cooled macaroons or store them in a tightly sealed container.

NUTRITION

Calories: 371.
Fat: 15 g.
Carbohydrates: 7 g.

Sugar: 2 g.
Protein: 41 g.
Cholesterol: 135 mg.

Conclusion

Did you see how you can prepare delicious and mouth-watering plant-based diet meals, and how easy the transition to a plant-based lifestyle can be? I hope you take the steps necessary to make the switch today. Do not be confused or disheartened by the misinformation that exists about plant-based diets. Now that you know better, you can take the steps necessary for changing your life and your diet. It ensures it will not be difficult or overly complicated. Take it one step and one recipe at a time, and go at a pace that is comfortable for you. Experiment with the recipes and come up with some of your own. Half the fun of the plant-based diet lifestyle is experimenting with your cooking skills.

With all these recipes here in this book, plus the tips given to you, I hope that you find the plant-based diet easy to follow. However, without commitment, it will be impossible for you to achieve your set goals. Develop a practical plan that will help you transition smoothly into the plant-based lifestyle. While doing this, you should also need that your environment is conducive to focusing on your diet plan. Your efforts should be directed towards learning more about the plant-based diet only.

When making a leap from other diets to plant-based diets, anything can happen along the way. Of course, there are instances where you might fall off the wagon and turn to animal-based diets or processed foods. However, what you should understand is that it is normal to fall and regress occasionally. The transformation is not easy; therefore, forgive yourself for making mistakes here and there. Concentrate on the bigger picture of living a blissful life where you are at a lower risk of cancer, diabetes, and other ailments. More importantly, keep yourself inspired by connecting with like-minded people. Do not overlook their importance in the transition, as they are also going through the challenge you are facing. Hence, they should advise you from time to time on what to do when you feel stuck.

Cheers to a healthy life! May you find the fulfillment of your goals through the plant-based diet movement!

Thank you for reading This book.
If you enjoyed it please visit the site where you
Purchased it and write a brief review. Your Feedback is important to me and will
help other readers decide whether to read the book too.
Thank You
Keli Bay

If you like reading diet books I have great news for you. You can download Keto Air Fryer
Desserts Cookbook for FREE simply by entering your name and email by visiting
www.topeditionltd.com/landing-page.